Raising Our Children Out of Poverty

Raising Our Children Out of Poverty has been co-published simultaneously as *Social Thought,* Volume 19, Number 2 1999.

Raising Our Children Out of Poverty

John J. Stretch
Maria Bartlett
William J. Hutchison
Susan A. Taylor
Jan Wilson
Editors

Raising Our Children Out of Poverty has been co-published simultaneously as *Social Thought,* Volume 19, Number 2 1999.

Routledge
Taylor & Francis Group
New York London

First published by

The Haworth Pastoral Press, 10 Alice Street, Binghamton, NY 13904-1580 USA

The Haworth Pastoral Press is an imprint of The Haworth Press, Inc., 10 Alice Street, Binghamton, NY 13904-1580 USA.

This edition published 2013 by Routledge

Routledge
Taylor & Francis Group
711 Third Avenue
New York, NY 10017

Routledge
Taylor & Francis Group
2 Park Square, Milton Park
Abingdon, Oxon OX14 4RN

Routledge is an imprint of the Taylor & Francis Group, an informa business

Raising Our Children Out of Poverty has been co-published simultaneously as *Social Thought,* Volume 19, Number 2 1999.

Cover design by Thomas J. Mayshock Jr.

Library of Congress Cataloging-in-Publication Data

Raising our children out of poverty / John J. Stretch . . . [et al.], editors.
p. cm.
"Co-published simultaneously as Social thought, volume 19, number 2 1999."
Includes bibliographical references and index.
ISBN 0-7890-0835-1 (alk. paper) – ISBN 0-7890-0845-9 (pbk: alk. paper)
1. Child welfare–United States–Congresses. 2. Poor children–United States–Congresses. 3. Poverty–United States–Congresses. 4. Church and social problems–Catholic Church–Congresses. 5. Church and social problems–United States–Congresses. I. Stretch, John J.

HV741 .R35 1999 99-046209

Raising Our Children Out of Poverty

CONTENTS

ABOUT THE EDITORS

John J. Stretch, PhD, MBA, ACSW, LCSW, is Professor of Social Work in the School of Social Service at Saint Louis University. He is a charter member of the Academy of Certified Social Workers and a Licensed Clinical Social Worker in the state of Missouri. Dr. Stretch is a nationally recognized social activist in the field of homelessness and housing. He has published extensively in major professional journals and books.

Maria Bartlett, PhD, is a former practitioner with over 15 years of experience in residential treatment, medical social work, and private practice. In 1990 she received a doctorate from the University of Illinois at Chicago. Her research interests include aging, health, feminist practice, international social work, and curriculum development. In 1992 she joined the faculty at Saint Louis University's School of Social Service and she has been a Center for Social Justice Advisory Board Member. As of 1999, she will teach in the Social Work Department at Humboldt State University, Arcata, California.

William J. Hutchison, PhD, is Associate Professor of Social Work in the School of Social Service at Saint Louis University. His areas of teaching include Social Welfare Policy and Spirituality, and Values and Religious Dimensions of Social Work. He serves on the Advisory Board of the Center for Social Justice Education and Research of the School of Social Service. From 1983 to 1993 he served as Dean of the School. He has published articles and book reviews in *Social Work* and *Social Thought: Journal of Religion in the Social Services.*

Susan A. Taylor, PhD, is Assistant Clinical Professor at the University of Denver Graduate School of Social Work. Dr. Taylor has been active in the social service and advocacy communities for two decades as a practitioner, policy analyst, and/or policy maker. Her commitment to low income and disenfranchised populations has been witnessed through her work and scholarship in areas of homelessness, poverty, AIDS, and disability. She has taught undergraduate and graduate Social Work at Saint Louis University School of Social Work, George Warren

Brown School of Social Work, Washington University, and the University of Denver Graduate School of Social Work. Her broad emphasis area is social welfare, family, and health policy. She most recently has chaired the children and family policy sequence at the University of Denver, and currently teaches in the policy and community practice areas.

Jan Wilson, MSW, LCSW, is a faculty liaison in the practicum program at Saint Louis University's School of Social Service, having joined the faculty in 1996. Her 25 years of professional experience include work as a therapist, program administrator, and community organizer. She has centered on services for families and children in child welfare, mental health, residential treatment, and school and community settings. Her interests also include consumer movements, inclusive programs for adults and children with developmental disabilities, health promotion for children and youth, and school social work. She serves on the Center for Social Justice Education Committee and chaired the Call for Papers for the 1998 Convening Conference.

Preface

As Editor of *Social Thought: Journal of Religion in the Social Services*, I am proud to bring to our readership this special volume on the social justice issues of children in poverty highlighted at the April, 1998 symposium, "Raising Children Out of Poverty." The symposium was sponsored by the Emmet and Martha Doerr Center for Social Justice, Education and Research, at Saint Louis University School of Social Service. This volume is particularly timely given the prevalence of poverty among children in the United States. Census Bureau statistics reveal that children under the age of eighteen had a significantly higher rate of poverty (19.9%) than their adult counterparts, aged eighteen to sixty-four (10.5%). Even though children make up only one-fourth of the total population, according to the Bureau, this group represents 40% of the poor population in the United States (Dalaker & Naifeh, 1997).

The journal *Social Thought* has a strong history of promoting social justice issues in keeping with social work values and ethics as well as Catholic social teaching. Its concern with poverty among families and children has been apparent from its inception as illustrated by Rev. Edward Ryle's article, "Poverty and Poor Relief in the United States: Two Interpretations and Some Implications," published in the inaugural issue, spring of 1975. Articles included in this volume discussing the future of foster care, ecumenical housing, collaborative practice in low-income communities, among others, continue this important tradition. Therefore, I would like to extend gratitude and thanks to the editors: John J. Stretch, PhD, MBA, ACSW, LCSW; Maria Bartlett, PhD; William J. Hutchison, PhD; Susan A. Taylor, PhD; and Jan Wilson, MSW, LCSW, who made this book possible.

Elizabeth D. Smith
Editor, Social Thought

REFERENCE

Dalaker, J., & Naifeh, M. U.S. Bureau of the Census, Current Population Reports, Series P 60-201, *Poverty in the United States: 1997*, U.S. Government Printing Office, Washington, DC, 1998.

Introduction

John J. Stretch
Susan A. Taylor

The test of any great society
is in how it treats its
most vulnerable.

–Hubert Humphrey

The papers selected for this special edition are from the April 1998 inaugural conference of the Emmet and Martha Doerr Center for Social Justice Education and Research. The Center, housed at the Saint Louis University School of Social Service, was designed to enhance the combined missions of excellence in education and commitment to social justice which are the fundamental cornerstones of both the School of Social Service and Saint Louis University. The Center's philosophy focuses upon six principles: (a) encouraging the education of the whole person; (b) promoting openness to seeking truth; (c) encouraging respect and appreciation for the uniqueness of each person; (d) celebrating diversity in cultural differences; (e) instilling a commitment to social justice among members of the social work practice and university communities; and (f) fostering a passion for the development of community initiatives which enhance the lives of the vulnerable. These contribute to the overlapping vision of Catholic social justice teaching and social work values and ethics.

The April symposium, "Raising Children Out of Poverty," reflects the Center's commitment to enlightening the discourse surrounding complex

John J. Stretch, PhD, is Professor of Social Work, School of Social Services, Saint Louis University, Saint Louis, MO.

Susan A. Taylor, PhD, is Assistant Professor, Barry University, School of Social Work, Miami, FL.

[Haworth co-indexing entry note]: "Introduction." Stretch, John J., and Susan A. Taylor. Co-published simultaneously in *Social Thought* (The Haworth Pastoral Press, an imprint of The Haworth Press, Inc.) Vol. 19, No. 2, 1999, pp. 1-5; and: *Raising Our Children Out of Poverty* (ed: John J. Stretch et al.) The Haworth Pastoral Press, an imprint of The Haworth Press, Inc., 1999, pp. 1-5. Single or multiple copies of this article are available for a fee from The Haworth Document Delivery Service [1-800-342-9678, 9:00 a.m. - 5:00 p.m. (EST). E-mail address: getinfo@haworthpressinc.com].

social issues faced by our society. The papers presented at the symposium reverberate the desire to promote socially responsible policy and practice methods, in conjunction with research and community empowerment models emphasizing the values of social work. An Editorial Board composed of policy/practice scholars associated with the Center reviewed the papers and selected ones which represented some of the best innovative thinking. The articles are a synergistic blend of critical thinking with respect to ethical and social policy issues affecting poor children and families, along with emerging conceptualizations of "best practice" models.

The conference was timely, as the nation is and has been engaged in reflecting anew as to its moral commitment to the nation's children–especially those who are the most vulnerable and dependent upon the whims of public policy. While media-savvy politicians have conveyed the highly racist and sexist image of poverty as an urban, black, and female single-parent problem, data rebuts this view. Rather, it reflects the underlying structural issues which are apparent in the poverty issue but missing from the public discourse. The Children's Defense Fund (CDF) (1998), for example, notes that three in five poor children are white; one in five lives in suburban America; one in three lives in a family with married parents; and two in three live in a working family (*The State of America's Children Yearbook,* 1998, p. xvii). Other data indicates that in spite of a thriving economy the rate of poverty is increasing. Census Bureau data reveals that "in 1973, 14.4% of all children in America were poor; by 1996 the rate had climbed to 20.5 percent. For young families . . . the child poverty rate doubled, from 20% in 1973 to 41% in 1994" (CDF, 1998, p. 3). Since the implementation of welfare reform in 1996, recent data has reflected a continued increase in child poverty. The Center for Children in Poverty (1998) reports a two-year increase in poverty among children in three of the most populous states–California, New York, and Texas. Likewise data from five smaller states–Oklahoma, Montana, Arizona, West Virginia, and Louisiana–show poverty increases among poor children from 40 to 53 percent (*News and Issues,* Summer/Fall 1998). Driven by political ideology and not social science data, there has been a profound shift in public social policy with as-yet-untested consequences of risks and impacts for children in poor families.

The free market solution–much touted in the 1994 Contract with America–appears to devalue human misery and encourage regressive public policy; seemingly reverting to an earlier Elizabethan poor law mentality of labeling the poor as lazy, shiftless, devoid of moral character, and requiring correction and transformation through work. Increasingly, private charity organizations– churches and social welfare agencies–are being called upon to pick up the social and economic costs of the structural realignment shifting from public responsibility for the poor to private.

The ethical dimensions supporting the proper role and responsibility of faith based and private charity are explored in this volume through the lead article by John Coleman S. J. entitled "Compassion, Solidarity, and Empowerment: The Ethical Contribution of Religion to Society." The thought-provoking analysis cogently speaks to conceptualizations of religious ethics which call people of faith toward advocating for economically and socially just policies and programs, thus leading to the inclusion of marginalized people. Offering a national and international perspective of faith based advocacy efforts, Father Coleman suggests that questions of justice and fairness are answered through values of compassion, solidarity, and empowerment. The ultimate goal, he suggests, is the creation of a compassionate and communal response.

Sunny Harris Rome and Evelyn Slaght offer a unique glimpse of the impact of the Personal Responsibility and Work Opportunity Act of 1996. Presenting a strong qualitative analysis which suggests that welfare reform may impact children adversely, the authors "assess the impact of welfare reform on foster care" (p. 22). This research adds to the developing body of knowledge on the dissonance between family maintenance and child welfare policies. The article also suggests the critical need for research models which capture the changing nature of income maintenance policies and their potential impact upon parallel systems (in this case, foster care placement rates). Systemic limitations which inform research and policy making are explored.

The first among the articles addressing "best practice models" is Michael Forster and Timothy Rehner's contribution entitled "Delinquency Prevention in Poor and At-Risk African-American Youth: A Social Work Practice Innovation." The article describes a multi-organization collaboration to address delinquency problems in a local public housing project in Mississippi. Forster and Rehner's work adds to the body of literature which encourages reflection on programs which are alternatives to incarceration. The need to highlight such programs is critical in light of Congressional policy initiatives such as H.R. 3 (1997 session) and S.10 (1998 session) which would open the way for more emphasis on imprisonment of juveniles and the weakening of laws which separate juveniles from the adult prison population. This type of policy shift negates a twenty-four year precedent of prevention and intervention as established under the Juvenile Justice and Delinquency Prevention Act of 1974 and subsequent amendments. Scholarly contributions such as the one by Forster and Rehner provide research to assist the advocacy and program communities seeking to temper the national trend toward excessively punitive juvenile policy initiatives regardless of offense.

Innovative community empowerment partnerships are highlighted in the article by Cathryne Schmitz entitled "Collaborative Practice in Low Income Communities: University, Agency, Public School Partnerships." In a policy environment which encourages charter schools as the panacea for offering meaningful educational alternatives to public schools, this article suggests that community-based family support centers attached to public schools can have a significant positive impact upon the lives of high risk children and families. This research adds valuable data to the slowly increasing body of literature which encourages the reemergence of community-based schools. These types of programs–which fell by the wayside during the Reagan Administration– once provided hope and stability in poor neighborhoods. Work by Schmitz and others may help to empower communities to move toward time-tested models which have proved effective despite the current proclivity to direct public education funds away from poor communities.

A strengths practice perspective is given concrete expression in Nancie Palmer's article "Fostering Resiliency in Children: Lessons Learned in Transcending Adversity." The article introduces readers to the Differential Resiliency Model (DRM) which the author first developed for use with adult children of alcoholics. Palmer suggests that the model is transferable to other populations as an alternative non-pathologizing method which seeks to empower what the literature has termed "at-risk" children and families. The article adds contrast to the clinical social work literature which has historically struggled with the use of the therapeutic models which pathologize rather than empower client strengths. Palmer's work is particularly poignant in offering an innovative alternative in this era of managed care where the temptation is to revert to the medical model for use in therapeutic intervention with poor and at-risk populations.

Finally, this volume ends with an article describing an innovative family support and empowerment program that has received national recognition for sustained results. In "Ecumenical Housing: Providing Housing and Services," Christopher Krehmeyer, Peter Salsich, and Cathryne Schmitz provide insight into how long-term investment is important in moving low income, young, single-parent families to self-sufficiency. The article highlights the events leading to the creation of the program, its service provisions, and research indicating program impact. The work highlights the unique perspectives of the three authors: the program's Executive Director (Krehmeyer), a social worker and long-time housing advocate; a founding member of the Board of Directors (Salsich), an attorney and law professor who has contributed much scholarship toward the issue of low-income housing; and an outside evaluator (Schmitz), who is sought out by many programs serving low income clients in the Saint Louis metropolitan area to provide meaningful evaluation and recommendations toward program improvements. The authors bring unique talents to this work, illuminating another "best practices" model for empowering low income populations.

Combined and standing alone these articles offer a valuable contribution to scholarly work which seeks to encourage a compassionate society through embracing each of its members with respect and meaningful opportunity. The editors of this volume, along with the Board of Directors of the Center for Social Justice Education and Research, and the Center's staff were honored to be asked to contribute their voices to the social discourse surrounding the deconstruction of the social welfare system and the impact upon vulnerable populations. We have been reminded in our work toward the conference convening and in the subsequent tasks associated with preparing manuscripts for publication, that there are many caring and compassionate individuals in the faith, social service, and academic communities who still believe in the innate goodness of each individual, the positive impact of caring supportive communities, and the need to stand in solidarity with those who are less fortunate than themselves. We thank them for their insights and contributions.

REFERENCES

Children's Defense Fund (1998). *The state of America's children yearbook.* Washington, DC: Children's Defense Fund.

The Center for Children in Poverty (Summer/Fall 1998). Child poverty in many states takes a turn–mostly for the worse. *News and Issues*, *8*(2), 1-2.

Compassion, Solidarity and Empowerment: The Ethical Contribution of Religion to Society

John A. Coleman S. J.

SUMMARY. This served as the Msgr. John Schoklee lecture in Social Justice and as a keynote for the conference "Raising Children Out of Poverty" at St. Louis University. The author argues that compassion, solidarity and empowerment represent the three key anchors of Catholic social teaching. All three are inter-related.

The concrete embodiment of compassion–so as to remove mere sentimental vagueness to the concept, entails the three-fold practices of direct social services, public advocacy and strategies of empowerment. In particular, the Catholic notion of justice as participation looks to the active empowerment of those who are marginalized. Ultimately, welfare means more than merely providing for those in need. It looks to enabling them to become active agents in society.

Having sketched the social teaching, the author then looks to sociological evidence about how well the churches practice what they preach. In our society, churches pre-eminently generate acts of compassion through voluntarism. Members of churches are more likely to give time and money to the voluntary sector than non-members. The paper ends with a sketch of one concrete program of empowerment: church-based community organizing. *[Article copies available for a fee from The Haworth Document Delivery Service: 1-800-342-9678. E-mail address: getinfo@haworthpressinc.com <Website: http://www.haworthpressinc.com>]*

KEYWORDS. Social ethics, social justice, social solidarity, voluntarism, faith-based organizations

John A. Coleman S. J. is Casassa Professor in Social Values, Loyola Marymount University, 7900 Loyola Boulevard, Los Angeles, CA 90045.

[Haworth co-indexing entry note]: "Compassion, Solidarity and Empowerment: The Ethical Contribution of Religion to Society." Coleman, John A. Co-published simultaneously in *Social Thought* (The Haworth Pastoral Press, an imprint of The Haworth Press, Inc.) Vol. 19, No. 2, 1999, pp. 7-20; and: *Raising Our Children Out of Poverty* (ed: John J. Stretch et al.) The Haworth Pastoral Press, an imprint of The Haworth Press, Inc., 1999, pp. 7-20. Single or multiple copies of this article are available for a fee from The Haworth Document Delivery Service [1-800-342-9678, 9:00 a.m. - 5:00 p.m. (EST). E-mail address: getinfo@haworthpressinc.com].

We ought to be as interested in what religion does as in what it says. For, religion enables and empowers just as much as it preaches and teaches. When we ask about the ethical contribution of religion to society, we should never forget, as Ernst Troeltsch states it in his classic study, *The Social Teachings of the Christian Churches*, that the church *is* and *enacts* a social ethic before it explicitly expounds one (Troetsch, 1960, I:90-196).

Moreover, it is perfectly possible for churches to empower even when they do not teach and to teach correctly but not empower. A sociologist at the University of California in Los Angeles, Stanley R. Bailey, is currently doing research in Brazil, comparing Pentecostal and Catholic parishes on the issue of racial empowerment. The Pentecostals do not much talk about race. They avoid any overt alliances with 'secular' black Brazilian groups working for racial justice. In their explicit teachings, they downplay mention of race. Brazilian Catholics, for their part, form coalitions with the secular Black movement for racial justice. The Brazilian bishops have written a strong and forthright pastoral letter condemning racism.

Yet, Bailey argues, at the local congregational level, the Pentecostals actually do more to integrate black members, enable them into leadership roles and empower them than do the local Catholic parishes which remain still rather white-dominated in their leadership structure. Without talking much about it, the Pentecostals are actually more effective than Catholics in empowering their black members.

I want to lift up three concepts which succinctly sum up religious ethics: compassion, solidarity and empowerment. For each I will ask: How does religion enact these in ways such that society is, thereby, ethically empowered ? These three are closely inter-related. They also rather clearly represent the three key components in a contemporary Catholic social ethic (Baum, 1989).

COMPASSION

All religions expect their devotees to be compassionate and to perform acts of compassion. I want to summarize, first, the major components of compassion as they appear in social Catholicism and, then, ask: How well do those who are religious in America actually perform acts of compassion? In two of his major social encyclicals, *Sollicitudo Rei Socialis* (1987) and *Centissimus Annus* (1991), John Paul II proposes compassion and solidarity as the two fundamental concepts to summarize and understand the tradition of Catholic social teaching.

To avoid being sentimental or merely preachy about compassion, Catholic social thinking has insisted that the church become involved at three distinct levels of compassion: (1) *Social Services*; (2) *Advocacy for Programs*; and (3) *Empowerment for the Powerless* (O'Brien and Shannon, 1992:42).

Social Services

In soup kitchens and Catholic Charities; in work dealing with undocumented refugees; in outreach in hospices and other services for those who suffer from AIDS; in community organizing programs in neighborhoods where people feel powerless about crime, drugs and the delivery of basic services; in its work with the unemployed and in counseling services–the church learns, *experientially*, that the present American society is not doing so well by its poor (Greider, 1992).

Direct contact through social service acts as a powerful corrective against turning the marginal members of the society into a mere statistic. Pedro Casadiglia, the poet bishop of Brazil, once said to a group of Indians in his society: "They make you an anonymous collective, without face or history." Direct social service guarantees that members of the church can give a face and history to those they serve. It shows an *immediate* compassion.

Advocacy for Programs

Yet, an important strategic move from initial compassion turns toward a less immediate structural analysis of poverty, unemployment, plant closings, lack of health care, etc. Since Vatican II, Catholics speak about structural sin or social sin. They mean by this that if you want to have true compassion for those in need, you can not simply put all your energy into emergency stop-gap solutions such as soup kitchens or houses for battered women. You need to address the larger structural issues which touch the economic, political and social health of our communities.

In order to engage in effective advocacy and lobbying, we have to do a social analysis and ask: What social structures cause these injuries to human dignity and what changes would be needed to provide humane basics for health care, food, education, housing, employment, family strength and community in our neighborhoods?

One of the strengths of the Catholic tradition of social thought lies in a certain humility when it comes to the concrete task of social analysis. The 'secular' retains its own rightful autonomy. Thus, we need to study as much as anyone else and, out of that study and joint discussion, we can propose tentative policy proposals. The gospel may tell us to say a loud *no*, in compassion, when we see human dignity infringed. It does not tell us, however, *how* to right the wrongs. This calls for study and dialogue. Again, as Troeltsch famously proclaimed: "Nowhere does there exist an absolute Christian ethic which only awaits discovery" (Troeltsch, 1960, II:1013).

Advocacy takes place through agencies such as Catholic Charities, the U.S. and State Catholic Conferences and in specialized lobby groups such as *Network*, *The Center of Concern* and other similar groups. To avoid superficiality, compassion must also embrace social analysis: systematic reflection on our lived experience. This is why social service and a university setting are so compatible. They need each other. Gustavo Guiterrez, the well-known Peruvian Liberation theologian, once put it this way: "We should avoid confusing gospel radicalness with intellectual laziness." Effective advocacy grows out of deep study and wrestling with the structures of society, the complexity of policy issues and the possibilities of our country. In a recent splendid book, *Catholic Social Teaching and United States Welfare Reform*, Thomas Massaro S.J. presents an exemplary case study of how to translate Catholic social thought into concrete policy for welfare reform (Massaro, 1998).

Empowerment

The third and final step to turn compassion into effectiveness lies in a strong conviction that real justice for those in need means that they must have some genuine sense of their own agency and participation in society. So, Catholic social thought is interested in strategies of empowerment.

Catholic social thought distinguishes three distinct forms of justice: (1) *Distributive Justice*, i.e., a fair method of sharing the 'common public' goods of society; (2) *Commutative Justice*, i.e., the justice involved in keeping contracts and promises; and (3) *Justice as Participation* (Hollenbach, 1988). Justice as participation rests on a key insight that the marginal members of society will have justice done and their dignity respected only when they can really actively participate and not just be recipients of other people's benevolence. It is not enough to provide for the needs of the poor if they remain mere passive recipients of aid. Here is how the American bishops put the point in their 1986 pastoral on economics:

> The prime purpose of this special commitment to the poor is to enable them to become active participants in the life of society. It is to enable *all* persons to share in and contribute to the common good. The 'option for the poor,' therefore, is not an adversarial slogan that pits one group or class against another. Rather it states that the deprivation and powerlessness of the poor wounds the whole community. The extent of their suffering is a measure of how far we are from being a true community of persons. (O'Brien and Shannon, 1992:600)

American Catholics have shown their concern for empowerment through the instrumentalities of church-based community organizing and *The Campaign for Human Development*. The ethical imperative to translate compassion into effective social service, advocacy and empowerment is quite clear. How effective, however, are the churches and synagogues in actually enacting compassionate social service?

THE CHURCHES AND SOCIAL CAPITAL

We have a great deal of sociological evidence about the relation of religion and compassion. Nancy Ammerman, in her national survey of congregations and parishes, *Congregation and Community*, notes:

> Our culture sees helping the needy as a religious virtue and expects religious organizations to be engaged in service activities. Part of the cultural definition that surrounds religious institutions is that they will provide direct services to people who need their help. That same cultural definition makes it likely that people in need will seek out congregations as sources of help.

Ammerman found that nearly all congregations report some form of direct human service activities, often through coalitions, rather than directly. The provision of social services congregations engage in is very broad. As Ammerman puts it: "[F]rom affordable housing to shelters for abused women, from food pantries, to refugee resettlement, congregations are often the organizational vehicles for the ameliorative work that needs to be done in a community" (Ammerman, 1997:366).

Case studies abound of church involvement in compassionate social service. The bulk of the feeding ministry in this country takes place through church coalitions. *Bread for the World*, a church-based lobby group, is the largest hunger advocacy group in the country. The homeless ministry is also mainly anchored in the churches. Much of the non-profit housing corporation-sector, building or rehabilitating affordable housing, are also religiously based (Fuller, 1994; Shabecoff, 1992). *Habitat for Humanity* is the largest of these groups. Religious organizations provide something like half or more of all the beds in AIDS hospices in this country.

After the communal uprising in South Central Los Angeles in the wake of the Rodney King verdict in 1992, the normal flow of food into the area was severely disrupted. Supermarkets had been burned and looted. The churches in the area, still standing, mobilized into action. They activated their food and clothing networks to do what even the government of the City of Los Angeles had neither contingency plans nor adequate resources to do. John Orr and his associates at the University of Southern California have studied this church response to urban crisis. They comment: "Inventories were already in place, volunteers were already recruited. The distribution sites were already identified–religious institutions located on almost every square mile of the affected area" (Orr, Miller, Roof, Melton, 1994). Orr points to what social scientists call 'social capital.'

I want to raise up this notion of social capital. Religion in America generates an inordinate amount of social capital. Social capital–a term made famous by Harvard political scientist Robert Putnam–points to communitarian features of social life, such as networks of mutuality and norms of trust, that enable participants to act together more effectively to pursue shared objectives. To the extent that social capital serves a bridging function–where norms, networks and trust link substantial sectors of the community and span underlying cleavages (e.g., of race and class)–social cooperation is enhanced and serves broader rather than narrower interests (Putnam, 1993, 1995).

Putnam links social capital to conventional political participation. While social capital is not exactly the same as political participation, it leads to and maximizes it. People connected to networks of communication and mutuality are more likely to vote and engage in volunteer civic activity. The renewal of an active citizenship in America, argues Putnam, must look especially to the renewal of social capital. Yet, no other institution in America generates as much social capital as the churches. People who are active in them are more apt to volunteer and to give money to the institutions of civil society–not just to churches–but to non-church activity (Hodgkinson, Weitzman, Kirch, 1988).

The churches regularly and straightforwardly act as communication networks that foster civic volunteerism. Princeton sociologist Robert Wuthnow puts it this way: "Religious organizations tell people of opportunities to serve, both within and beyond the congregation itself, and provide personal contacts, committees, phone numbers, meeting space, transportation or whatever it may take to help turn good intent into action" (Wuthnow, 1994a:242).

The sociological evidence linking religion to social capital seems overwhelming. Two-thirds of those active in social movements in America (even secular-sounding ones) claim that they draw on religious motivation for their involvement. In my own study of six citizen-activist groups in America, I found the majority of respondents gave religious motivation as their primary reason for being involved in hunger ministries, building low-cost housing for the poor, being engaged in peace activism, etc. (Coleman, 1996; 1998). Two-thirds of all small support groups in America are directly connected with churches and synagogues (Wuthnow, 1994b). As Wuthnow has put it, in his national study of student volunteers in America, "Churches and synagogues remain the primary place where instruction is given about the spiritual dimension of caring" (Wuthnow, 1995:9). Wuthnow elaborates his point: "The social ethos of the churches may be as important, if not more so, as a stimulus to volunteerism, as is the specific content of religious teachings"

(Wuthnow, 1995:267). To make caring through volunteerism meaningful, some framework of interpretation is required. Churches provide that framework. Church-sponsored volunteerism, as Wuthnow also claims, is associated with a feeling that one can make a difference in society. In short, voluntarism empowers people to act (Wuthnow, 1995:283).

Americans give seven times as much to churches as to political campaigns and several times as much as they give to secular charities. They also seem to think that churches and synagogues are better able to deal with "the problems facing our city or local community." Fifty-seven percent of respondents, in one Gallop survey, deemed churches to be more apt to deal with such problems than other institutions. Less than a third thought local business, government or political parties were apt vehicles for compassionate and just solutions to the problems of our local communities (*Emerging Trends,* 1990).

People are more likely to give time and money, even to secular efforts, if they are church members. They are also significantly more likely to vote if they are church members. In his study of volunteers in America, Wuthnow discovered that religiously motivated volunteers were also more likely than were the non-religious to employ a communitarian language and appeal to some sense of the common good, rather than to appeal to merely individualistic language, to explain their behavior (Wuthnow, 1991:325). Another study shows that even having neighbors who attend church is a critical factor in predicting whether youths in a neighborhood will have jobs, use drugs or engage in criminal activity. The social capital of churches spills over into whole neighborhoods (Case and Katz, 1991). Glenn Loury has noted that "the reports of successful efforts at reconstruction in ghetto communities invariably reveal a religious institution or a set of devout believers at the center of the effort" (Schambra, 1994:32).

THE CHURCHES AND CIVIC VOLUNTEERISM

In their massive study of political and civic volunteerism in America, Sidney Verba, Kay Schlozman and Henry Brady argue that religion significantly increases the democratic potential of the United States. Along with the workplace and non-political civic organizations, such as the Rotary Club, churches offer three important resources that increase the likelihood and effectiveness of both civic and political involvement:

1. They train people in transferable skills, such as giving a speech, organizing a meeting, writing a memo or raising money–skills that can then be translated into a wider citizenship activism.

2. They provide dense networks from which civic activists can be recruited. People respond better to requests for activity when asked by a friend rather than a stranger.
3. They give people a sense of efficacy in a local setting which, in turn, increases the chances they will feel that they actually can have some real impact in the public sphere.

The workplace has a built-in bias toward providing these civic and political advantages to the affluent and well-educated. Those who already have, receive even more. Nor does the corporate workplace overcome these biases. Managers, rather than ordinary workers, are routinely asked to organize the meetings, write the memos and give the speeches. The same is true of non-religious civic organizations. Verba, Schlozman and Brady discovered, almost to their surprise, that among major American institutions, only churches compensated by making democracy more representative, in giving the voiceless skills and voice.

They conclude their study with these remarks: "Only the religious institutions provide a counter-balance in this cumulative resource process. They play an unusual role in the American participatory system by providing opportunities for the development of civic skills to those who would be otherwise resource poor" (Verba, Schlozman, Brady, 1995:18-19). Indeed, a blue collar worker in America is more apt to be given opportunities to practice civic skills in church than in a union, "not because American unions are particularly deficient as skill builders but because so few American blue-collar workers are union members and so many are church members" (Verba, Schlozman, Brady, 1995:520). Thus, a working-class deacon in the black church receives organizing and communication skills beyond what his job would provide. The churches make our society more participatory, more egalitarian and more communitarian than it would be without them.

SOLIDARITY

Along with compassion, solidarity is the second major lens to see Catholic social teaching. How can we become more aware of our interdependent world? John Paul II has made the term "solidarity" central to the Catholic social vision. Here is how he describes it:

> Solidarity helps us to see the other–whether a person, people or nation–not just as some kind of instrument, with a work capacity and physical strength to be exploited at low cost and then discarded when no longer useful, but as a neighbor, a helper (cf. Gen. 2:18-20), to be made a sharer, on a par with ourselves, in the banquet of life to which all are equally invited by God. (O'Brien and Shannon, 1992:423)

The sociological evidence is more spotty–because less systematic–about how religion generates a greater solidarity. In my own interviews with 400 respondents engaged in citizen-activist movements, I asked them to state how they conceptualized citizenship. Rather typically I heard responses which, on a religious ground, expanded the notion of citizenship to a much larger solidarity. Let the following two voices be representative. The founder of *Habitat for Humanity*, Millard Fuller, told me in his interview: "I wear my citizenship in the United States very lightly because there is a citizenship greater than being a U.S. citizen." A Detroit *Bread for the World* member echoes this same theme: "We are citizens of the world and not just of the United States."

EMPOWERMENT AND CHURCH-BASED COMMUNITY ORGANIZING

One of the citizenship groups I studied, *PICO* (an acronym for the *Pacific Institute of Community Organizing*), is one of the four largest national church-based community organizing groups. Community organizing can represent for us an important case study of how religion empowers ordinary citizens.

Listen, at the outset, to some voices from my interviews. In Pensacola, church leaders storm the police chief's office, demanding action to clean up drug use in crack houses and on-the-street drug dealing which has left the elderly prisoners in their own homes. Willie May Randerson gave us this account of her meeting with the Pensacola police chief:

> We had called for an appointment to come in and they kept giving us the runaround. So finally fifteen of us loaded into our cars and went down. We asked to see the chief of police, we are taxpayers and have a right to see him. He sends in another person to tell us the chief is busy–he doesn't have time to see us. These people in the neighborhood pay the same taxes as the people in the upper-class neighborhood of the city and I told him we were going to sit and we were not going to move until we saw the chief of police.
>
> After 45 minutes, he came out and he opened the door and told us to come in. He wanted to know why there were so many of us. By then, the Christian that I am is speaking to me and says: Peace be still! I told him: "Why are there so many? Look here. We have fifteen people here, some is sixty and Miss Mccannako is 93 years old. Some's fat and some's skinny; some's pretty and some's ugly. Am I supposed to weed them out and say: 'You can't go because of your age?' When you get ready to get your salary from these people's property, you don't tell

> them that they don't have to pay taxes because they are too old. For that reason, we all have a right to be here." Then we quietly sat down, with the eight chairs he provided. The others of us just stood and he says "well, if you don't sit, you won't stay long" and I told him that the Lord was going to hold us up and we didn't have to sit. He's going to be our prop if we have to stand so let's get on with what we came here to talk about.

The group lodges its complaint that, when a call about a burglary or drug abuse in their neighborhood comes into the police communication center, it takes three or four hours before they dispatch a deputy to cover it. In upper class neighborhoods, they had learned, a deputy is speedily sent out within fifteen minutes. Their intervention is successful. The police chief is won over and the police protection gets provided.

Church-based community organizing in this country remains the great untold story of faith-based civic activism and empowerment. It numbers approximately three million adherents (compare this to the 1.7 million in the Christian Coalition which gets so much more press) and has strong potentiality for renewing our democratic citizenship.

The scene we witnessed above is not isolated. In New Orleans, some 6000 people come together, under the aegis of a federation of Protestant, Catholic and Jewish congregations, led by a black minister, demanding draconian police reform to halt endemic police corruption. In New Orleans, they successfully achieve their goal that the two major candidates for mayor commit, in advance of the election, in the company of the new city cabinet, to a full-day meeting with representatives of the church-based organizing group to discuss specific plans for reforming the police department and cleaning up (by rehabilitation or removal) of thousands of abandoned houses in the center city. The church group, in its mission statement, declares as one of its goals:

> *Pico* views accountability as the key missing ingredient in public life. It is the iron rule of *Pico*. Accountability is at the core of a democratic society. It is too precious to be left to election time alone. It must be acted on throughout the life of a public servant and to be expected in public office. Without accountability, distrust exists. The hope that the quality of life can improve and the fabric of our communities be rewoven can exist only when trust is real and not a slogan.

Pico now has 400 local organizing units, extending from the west coast, to the south, midwest and New Jersey, New York and Pennsylvania. The congregations and parishes belonging to *Pico* span 26 different Christian and Jewish religious congregations: Catholic, mainline Protestant, the black churches and evangelicals. The racial breakdown of *Pico* members is 37.7%

Anglo; 22.5% African-American; 31.8% Hispanic; 7.5% Asian. The gender breakdown of groups and staff is roughly equal male and female. Few other American organizations so span the racial, class and religious divides in our country, bringing groups together and bridging the culture wars.

THE BRIDGING FUNCTION OF SOCIAL CAPITAL

Pico seems to have escaped the 'so-called' culture wars. It appeals beyond liberals and radicals. Sometimes the very first action people ask for in their neighborhoods is to clean up prostitution or pornography. There are close affinities between community organizing and the home-spun self-help tradition. The Reverend Paul Bryant, a Southern Baptist minister in Pensacola, told us:

> See, the ironic thing is I'm conservative, biblically, politically and you usually don't see that kind of bird involved in this type of work. But I believe we have to avail ourselves of this model. This is not something for the left or the right. I say that really, you take the churches out of this part of town, there's no voice for the people or with the people.

Contrast Bryant's testimony to the more participant democratic and radical populist vision of Mary Ellen Burton-Christie, a leader in the Oakland Federation with a background in the radical *Catholic Worker* tradition of Dorothy Day. She reflects on this more radical, populist strand in *Pico*:

> I think there was a time when singing God Bless America would make me ill, but if we had an action and sang it together, it would make me cry because of who was singing it and because of how much they meant it and because it wouldn't be God Bless America instead of everybody else. It would be God be with us in our lives, we need you here. I am not usually very sympathetic to the patriotic kinds of things, although I think organizing is a very patriotic thing to do. I think that being active in a democracy is very patriotic. We are being active participants in a democracy. That means a lot more to me now than it did 10 years ago. To me, being democratic meant I had to vote. Well, now to me, if somebody's just voting, they are barely doing what they need to do.

One of the major interests in this case is that community organizing began as a purely secular model which underwent important changes when community organizing moved from neighborhoods to churches as the primary base for its social location. Earlier, Alinsky-style organizing had often been, uncivilly, gruff and confrontational. It lacked, at times, any sense of genuine partnership between elected officials and corporations. When neighborhood issues got won, the organization, lacking a deeper bonding beyond mere issues, fell apart. Nor did the Alinsky model have a deep value-base on which to build. Alinsky, himself, found, to his chagrin, this value weakness in his technique. People he earlier organized in Chicago's Back of the Stockyards neighborhood actually used the same skills at organizing they had learned from him to keep blacks out of their neighborhood (Alinsky, 1969; Bailey, 1974)!

One of the community organizers we interviewed in Denver had started his career with the older Alinsky model. He elaborates on the theme of an ethical value-base and links it to the notion of religion's power in generating social capital:

> They [the churches] provide more of the long term vision and guidance and stability to the organization because the congregations are much more stable than the organization because they have been there for years. It gives you an incredibly strong courtroom when a local congregation decides to organize, because you might start with 15 or 20 people who are already in relationship and that have trust and commitment. They go out and bring people in who don't go to church here but what is so nice is that you've got these fifteen to twenty people that already trust one another and are in relationship and the problems the neighborhood organizing has where people start having turf battles with one another are not present. Here the new people kind of integrate into an already committed and developed group of leaders that are working together in love and respect. The congregation provides that. Then, the other thing is the congregation provides a whole new sense of self-interest. That is self-interest plus self-sacrifice. Other organizations that are issue-oriented only all operate on personal selfishness as a self-interest but congregations have this somewhat broader self-interest. Finally, congregation-based organizing is based on values and on principles and that's really important because it is able to look at questions of justice and fairness.

Religiously motivated citizens, we heard over and over again in our interviews, say they "are in it for the long haul." They want to win on an issue and make a difference, of course. But, in the end, they also want to bear witness to what they see as the truth, even when or if they are not winning.

When we put together compassion, solidarity and empowerment we have a strong recipe for a more communal and just society. But the religious roots are important. We asked Mary-Ellen Burton-Christie whether she thought she could be as good an organizer as she was without being religious. Her response can represent the last word to our topic of compassion, solidarity and empowerment:

No, I don't think I could. I think that when we organize, I think people really do feel like they are opening up and letting God work through them. I think there are a lot of people who are really serious about that. It sounds simple to say that your faith makes a difference but I think that's one way you hang on to hope. I hear so many stories [from other leaders] like that and how you can continue to be hopeful [even when things are not going well]. But somehow I do, and it's not because I think that things are going to get better fast. I think it's because I think there is a God. I think there is a God.

REFERENCES

Alinsky, Saul 1969. *Rules for Radicals* New York: Random House.

Ammermann, Nancy 1997. *Congregation and Community* New Brunswick: Rutgers University Press.

Bailey, Robert 1974. *Radicals in Urban Politics: The Alinsky Approach* Chicago: University of Chicago Press.

Baum, Gregory 1989. *Compassion and Solidarity: The Church for Others* Mahwah, New Jersey: Paulist Press.

Case, Anne and Katz, Lawrence, 1991. "The Company You Keep: Effects of Family and Neighborhood on Disadvantaged Youths," Cambridge, Mass.: National Bureau of Economic Research, Working Paper 3705.

Coleman, John 1996. "Under the Cross and the Flag," *America* May 11:6-14.

Coleman, John 1998. "Religion and Public Life: Some American Cases," *Religion* 28 (April 1988):155-69.

Emerging Trends 1990. "Churches Rated Best Able to Deal With Local Community Problems" Dec.:3-4.

Fuller, Millard 1994. *The Theology of the Hammer* Macon, Georgia: Smyth and Helwys Publishing Inc.

Greider, William 1992. *Who Will Tell the People?* New York: Simon and Schuster.

Hodkingson, Virginia, Weitzman, Murray and Kirch, Arthur 1988. *From Belief to Commitment: The Activities and Finances of Religious Congregations in the United States* Washington, D.C.: Independent Sector.

Hollenbach, David 1988. *Justice, Peace and Human Rights* New York: Crossroad.

Massaro, Thomas 1998. *Catholic Social Teaching and United States Welfare Reform* Collegeville, Minn: Liturgical Press.

O'Brien, David and Shannon, Thomas, eds. 1992. *Catholic Social Thought: The Documentary Heritage* Maryknoll, New York: Orbis Press.

Orr, John, Miller, Donald, Roof, Wade and Melton, J. Gordon 1994. *Politics of the Spirit: Religion and Multi-Ethnicity in Los Angeles* Los Angeles: University of Southern California.

Putnam, Robert 1995. "Bowling Alone Revisited," *The Responsive Community*: 18-33.

Schambra, William 1994. "The Old Values and the New Citizenship," *Policy Review* Summer: 32.

Shabecoff, Alice 1992. *Rebuilding Our Communities: How Churches Can Provide Support and Finance Quality Housing* Monrovia, Calif.: World Vision.

Troeltsch, Ernst 1960. *The Social Teachings of the Christian Churches* vols. 1 and 2 New York: Harper and Row.

Verba, Sidney, Schlozman, Kay and Brady, Henry 1995. *Voice and Equality* Cambridge, Mass: Harvard University Press.

Wuthnow, Robert 1991. *Acts of Compassion* Princeton: Princeton University Press.

1994a *God and Mammon in America* New York: The Free Press.

1994b *Sharing the Journey* New York: The Free Press.

1995 *Learning to Care* New York: Oxford University Press.

Welfare Reform and the Future of Foster Care

Sunny Harris Rome
Evelyn F. Slaght

SUMMARY. In an effort to document the impact of the Personal Responsibility and Work Opportunity Act of 1996 on the lives of children, the authors conducted a study in Washington, D.C. and the adjacent states of Maryland and Virginia. Interviews with key informants indicate that there is little quantitative data available, even in states like Virginia where recipients are reaching the 2-year time limit. In Maryland, data are only available on those leaving welfare early, and the impact there on the child welfare system is reported as "minimal." Focus of the data is on employment success, and evades the effects of low wages, inadequate child care availability, teen parenting issues, kinship care, and inadequate services, especially for those with substance abuse, health and mental health problems. Although quantitative data are limited, qualitative data indicate that the mandate of "personal responsibility" may become a mechanism for revoking our social commitment to protect children. *[Article copies available for a fee from The Haworth Document Delivery Service: 1-800-342-9678. E-mail address: getinfo@haworthpressinc.com <Website: http://www.haworthpressinc.com>]*

KEYWORDS. Welfare reform, foster care, child welfare, day care, poverty

---

Sunny Harris Rome, MSW, JD, is Assistant Professor and Evelyn F. Slaght, MSW, PhD, is Associate Professor, George Mason University (GMU), Fairfax, VA.

The authors wish to acknowledge the assistance of Ms. Beth Funk, social work student at GMU.

[Haworth co-indexing entry note]: "Welfare Reform and the Future of Foster Care." Rome, Sunny Harris, and Evelyn F. Slaght. Co-published simultaneously in *Social Thought* (The Haworth Pastoral Press, an imprint of The Haworth Press, Inc.) Vol. 19, No. 2, 1999, pp. 21-36; and: *Raising Our Children Out of Poverty* (ed: John J. Stretch et al.) The Haworth Pastoral Press, an imprint of The Haworth Press, Inc., 1999, pp. 21-36. Single or multiple copies of this article are available for a fee from The Haworth Document Delivery Service [1-800-342-9678, 9:00 a.m. - 5:00 p.m. (EST). E-mail address: getinfo@haworthpressinc.com].

INTRODUCTION

As states rush to demonstrate compliance with the Personal Responsibility and Work Opportunity Act of 1996 (PRWORA or P.L. 104-193), questions are being raised regarding the impact of this new policy on the lives of children. Many fear that, in the process of replacing AFDC with TANF, the historical emphasis on child protection will be lost in the interest of achieving "self sufficiency" through parental employment.

Current child welfare policy assumes that many families at-risk can be preserved through services that improve parenting (including protective services [CPS] and family preservation programs), and financial assistance that provides the fiscal safety net to avert foster care by meeting basic tangible needs.

Because of its new constraints on the receipt of financial assistance, there is reason to believe that welfare reform will have an adverse impact on children. Yet those who question the new policy are finding it difficult to document that mandatory work requirements and time limits on receipt of benefits are having any negative impact. Failure to generate data that can allow us to accurately document outcomes will prevent policy makers from making necessary adjustments to welfare policy, programs, or services.

In order to help assess the impact of welfare reform on foster care, the authors conducted a pilot study in Washington, D.C. and the adjacent states of Maryland and Virginia. The intent was to collect the available data on welfare reform, as well as information regarding the extent to which an impact on child welfare is being observed or anticipated.

LITERATURE REVIEW

It is widely agreed that children cannot be protected from maltreatment without guaranteeing basic economic support for families (Courtney, 1997). Whether or not the PRWORA will accomplish this goal remains a matter of controversy. Both the stringent work requirements and the limits on financial assistance have the potential to hinder the ability of some parents to care for their children (Bratz & White, 1996).

Under the PRWORA's predecessor, the Family Support Act, a connection was reported between the welfare experience and involvement with the child welfare system. A study in Los Angeles (Collins & Aber, 1998), for example, reported an increase in child abuse and neglect referrals following AFDC grant reductions. A study in Michigan found that sanctioned families in the JOBS program were more likely than other AFDC families to have contact with Child Protective Services (CDF, 1998). Data reported by the Urban Institute (Pavetti et al., 1997) indicate that recipients who did not respond to sanctions were more likely to experience "personal and family challenges" such as chemical dependency, mental health and health problems.

An even more dramatic effect is predicted under the PRWORA. According to Geen and Waters (1997), if the economic well-being of families worsens, abuse and neglect are likely to increase. This is supported by recent data from the Children's Defense Fund (1998) showing a 25% increase in the number of children in foster care between 1990 and 1996. Since the foster care program is an outgrowth of AFDC and about half of the children in care come from welfare dependent families (Courtney, 1995), policies that further jeopardize family financial resources are likely to impact the child welfare system even further. "Child protection caseloads may increase when families, under additional financial stress, commit more child abuse and neglect or voluntarily place their children in foster care" (Hardin, 1997, p. 1068).

The children who are most vulnerable to involvement with the child welfare system under welfare changes include the following (Knitzer & Bernard, 1998):

- children whose families are sanctioned
- children whose families reach the time limits
- children in families where economic hardship leads to maltreatment
- children no longer eligible for SSI
- children of legal immigrants who lose benefits
- children now in kinship foster care
- children in care where work requirements interfere with reunification
- youth "aging out" of the foster care system

Although welfare reform has made additional funds available to meet its adult-focused goals (Collins & Aber, 1998), child welfare agencies are likely to emerge with fewer, rather than more, resources. In addition to reductions in federal funding for services to abused and neglected children (Videka-Sherman & Viggiani, 1996), new cutbacks in funding for the Title XX Social Services Block Grant are expected to strain agency resources, limiting opportunities for much needed prevention activities (Geen & Waters, 1997).

Those who are anticipating the outcomes of federal policy changes caution that we must go beyond simply counting employment successes as we seek to understand the full impact of welfare reform (Videka-Sherman &Viggiani, 1996). As Courtney (1995) points out, failure to attend to the consequences of welfare reform for the foster care program is "a serious and potentially expensive oversight" (p. 27).

METHODOLOGY

In order to further existing efforts to document the consequences of welfare reform for children and the child welfare system, the authors interviewed key informants in the District of Columbia, Maryland, and Virginia. These three geographic areas represent considerable diversity in terms of demographics, urban/rural/suburban settings, political orientation, and welfare reform implementation strategies.

Our informants, including researchers and planners at the state level as well as local child welfare program managers, supervisors and line staff, were first asked to provide data on how welfare reform had affected foster care rates. It quickly became apparent that there were limited data available, but our study would nonetheless be valuable if it could identify data needs, obstacles to data collection, and potential ways to overcome these obstacles. Informants were questioned about their observations and subjective expectations regarding any potential impact of welfare reform on their agencies or clients. They were asked to describe any planning efforts underway to ready the agency for the possible repercussions of welfare reform, and to discuss their hopes and concerns about the well-being of children and families under the new law.

FINDINGS

Quantitative Data

Extensive efforts were undertaken to identify existing empirical data on the implications of welfare reform. While most jurisdictions reported high rates of job placement, few were able to document a relationship between employment and child well-being. The most common response of the jurisdictions to our inquiries was that most of the clients affected by work requirements are getting jobs. Maryland, through a partnership between the State Department of Human Resources (DHR) and the University of Maryland School of Social Work (UMSSW), has been able to track families as they exit welfare. Of the 1216 children whose families exited welfare between October, 1996 and September, 1997, only four children (from two families) came into foster care. All of these families exited before reaching the mandated time limits. The study concludes that the impact of welfare reform on foster care at this time is minimal. It should be noted, however, that those leaving welfare during this one-year period were those with wage histories and work experience, making it more predictable that they would have a positive job experience (C. Born, personal communication, February 11, 1998). Other recipients (including those with serious mental illness, physical disabilities, or substance abuse problems), who are more likely to stay on the rolls until they exhaust their benefits, were not included in this study. These are the families that are most likely to require CPS or foster care services, even if they ultimately succeed in entering jobs.

Like Maryland, the other two jurisdictions pointed out that, even though many welfare clients are having success at this point, entry into employment alone is not expected to insure against negative family outcomes in the future. Because of the diversity of the welfare population, some will be well served by the new emphasis on employment, while others (including those with little education, substance abuse problems, criminal records, no work experience, or emotional problems) will require more support and be more difficult to sustain in the mainstream economy.

The three jurisdictions studied were also able to provide data regarding recent trends in foster care. Although these trends may not reflect the implementation of welfare reform, they give us a baseline against which to measure a possible future impact. Generally speaking, all report that the steady increase in foster care experienced throughout the 1980s and early 1990s has leveled off in the past two years–with the notable exception of the cities, where the number of children in foster care has continued to rise.

In Maryland, DHR data indicate that, in the past year, foster care caseloads have levelled off EXCEPT in Baltimore City where the growth is "explosive" (C. Cooper, personal communication, March 11, 1998). Records show 500 new foster care placements this year in addition to the 8500 children already in substitute care (in a city of approximately 700,000). The increase is not attributed to welfare reform, but rather to the increasing substance abuse problem in the city.

Likewise, the only urban center in Virginia, Richmond, has the largest foster care caseload in that state. Interviews with child welfare staff suggest that substance abuse is the major factor accounting for this phenomenon. Some suburban and rural areas report being affected by drug use, but it has not yet reached the epidemic levels that urban centers continue to experience. The only substance abuse problem reported in one small rural area in Virginia, for example, was parents misusing their children's Ritalin. On the other hand, one informant reported that, in her small jurisdiction, there is an upswing in substance abuse that appears to be linked to the relocation of a major employer in the area and a subsequent increase in unemployment.

Despite the availability of reliable data on both foster care rolls and early welfare reform efforts, little is known about the actual effects of benefit loss on children and families. For one thing, meaningful findings are largely premature. At the time the study was conducted, in two of the three jurisdictions (Maryland and D.C.) no clients had reached the time limit on receipt of TANF benefits. In the third (Virginia), because of a phased-in implementation and a 2-year (rather than 5-year) time limit, clients in some counties had already exhausted their benefits, although those in the most heavily populated counties were only beginning to do so. Although all three jurisdictions were collecting data regarding clients who voluntarily left the rolls, it was too soon to gauge the effects of forced benefit terminations under the new time limits on TANF receipt.

Even once the time limits are reached, it will take some time before any impact on child welfare–particularly foster care–can be discerned. If there are later contacts with the child welfare agency, they would not necessarily follow swiftly upon the heels of benefit termination. Neglect, in particular, often materializes gradually and takes time to be reported. Once a family does come to the attention of the child welfare system, foster care is unlikely to become an issue until interventions aimed at salvaging the family unit have proven unsuccessful. Consequently, identifying the impact of benefit terminations on foster care is necessarily a long-term proposition.

In addition, data collection efforts, generally, are in disarray (Vobejda & Havemann, 1998). In particular, many areas lack effective systems to track TANF recipients. Virginia, for example, is currently transitioning between information systems and is experiencing lengthy delays in its data collection efforts. One of its largest and most affluent counties still collects data manually. The District of Columbia's child welfare system, which is under a court-ordered receivership, operates entirely separately from its welfare department; hence, monitoring clients across agencies is a formidable task, and one which is not now being attempted.

These and other obstacles to the collection of empirical data on the link between welfare reform and child welfare point to the need for supplementary information that can shed light on the actual experience of families in the service system.

QUALITATIVE DATA

Because of the paucity of data available at the time of the study to document any impact of welfare reform on child welfare, efforts were made to acquire qualitative information through interviews. Again, little conclusive information was forthcoming. The reason, it seems, is that most agencies at both the state and local level are so preoccupied with implementing welfare reform that they have not yet turned their attention to positioning their child welfare agencies to handle any possible repercussions. Most of the staff are very optimistic about welfare reform and are focusing intently on efforts to move TANF recipients into the workplace; they are so committed to making welfare reform work that they are reluctant to consider what the fallout might be, in the event of failure. The reality, of course, is that no matter how successfully welfare reform is implemented, at least some families will end up suffering financial losses that could ultimately harm their children.

A common concern was the disconnect between staff responsible for welfare reform and those in child welfare. In many agencies there is little if any communication between the two and a striking lack of familiarity with the other's constraints and responsibilities. Child welfare workers, in particular, often demonstrated very limited understanding of the Personal Responsibility Act and how it was being implemented in their jurisdiction. Some were unable even to fathom the possibility of collaboration around addressing a particular family's needs.

In addition to interagency problems, the following were identified as areas of concern.

Child Care

Inadequate child care was a major issue identified by child welfare staff in all three jurisdictions. They anticipate that quality, availability, and affordability of care will adversely affect family well-being in the long run.

In the District of Columbia, under general receivership, the administrative and physical separation of the foster care system from the income maintenance agency has resulted in a lack of available child care funds to assist with family reunification or to support foster parents who work. Mothers who are newly employed and simultaneously reassuming their parental roles and responsibilities are likely to be overwhelmed under these conditions, yet the general receiver cannot assure them that child care will be available.

The problems of child care are most severe in relation to infants and children with special needs. According to a survey conducted by the Child Welfare League of America (1997), only 51% of the 41 states responding have opted to exempt parents of children under age one from the PRWORA's work requirement. This suggests that, nationally, the demand for infant care will be enormous, posing a formidable challenge in many states.

Another phenomenon relates to older children being left in charge of younger siblings, while their parents work multiple or non-traditional ("graveyard shift") jobs. Many mothers who cannot afford child care, or who face long waiting lists, feel pressured to take jobs they would not otherwise take, leaving their children improperly supervised. One Virginia county reported a mother feeling compelled to leave her 14-year-old daughter in charge of a younger brother with severe attention deficit hyperactivity disorder (ADHD), night after night, while she held down a job. She felt this was a better alternative than leaving the brother in her daughter's care during the daytime when he was awake and more difficult to control. Other parents of children with disabilities have reported being in a similar bind, feeling pressured to work (so as not to be sanctioned and risk loss of TANF benefits) despite the shortage of specialized child care resources. Some children are reporting going to sleep armed with baseball bats, terrified that intruders will enter while their parents are out working the night shift.

Lack of adequate resources, coupled with the pressure to work, has led some agencies to encourage families to seek informal care from relatives, friends, or neighbors. Agency staff, however, are apprehensive about the risk that this can entail, since these providers are unknown to the agency and may be unskilled, unreliable, abusive, or dangerous.

One county reported that, if the existing neglect statutes were strictly enforced, their child welfare agency would be overrun with cases because of the increasing incidence of inadequate supervision, brought about by the pressure to work. They have asked the state to consider easing their legal definition of "neglect" to keep these cases from entering the system.

Wages

Child welfare agency staff in all three jurisdictions also expressed concern that the incomes of those moving off the TANF rolls will be too low to enable them to support their families in the long run. Many recognize that strong state and local economies are currently favorable; they worry about what will happen in a weaker economy with fewer jobs and depressed wages.

A number of local jurisdictions have made special efforts to move TANF recipients into jobs paying more than the minimum wage. One of Virginia's affluent suburban counties, for example, boasts an average wage for former TANF recipients of $8.45 per hour. The problem is that even this amount is inadequate, given the high cost of living in an area where the average housing rental is $500-600 per month. While the median monthly income of former TANF recipients is $1,160, the median monthly income among the county's residents overall is $5,800. The concern is that people are indeed earning more, but not enough to move them out of poverty (Brown, 1998). Agency staff are concerned that many clients will earn too much to qualify for subsidies, but will earn too little to be financially stable.

This is compounded by the rules governing transitional child care benefits which, under federal law, continue for 12 months after a client moves off the TANF rolls and into a job. For many clients, wages will be inadequate to ensure the continued support of their families, especially once their transitional child care benefits are exhausted and child care expenses are added to their financial obligations. If clients are terminated from the TANF rolls but still cannot support their families, we again face the possibility of inadequate resources leading to neglect, and ultimately to substitute care.

Teen Parents

The fate of teenage parents is another area of concern raised by child welfare personnel. Federal law requires that, in order to be eligible for cash benefits, teen parents reside with a parent (or other adult) and attend school.

Recognizing that many teen parents come from abusive home situations, limited exceptions are permitted. Unfortunately, only 38% of states involve their child protective services staff in decision-making around the appropriate housing situation for their teenage welfare recipients (CWLA, 1997). This failure to collaborate may lead to poor outcomes for teens and their children who move into unsafe environments or who suffer financial sanctions for refusing to do so.

Personal Responsibility

One effect that welfare reform is already having on child welfare in some agencies is the adoption of a widespread philosophy of "personal responsibility." One Virginia county, in particular, has decided to promote personal responsibility throughout all facets of its social services department. Welfare reform clients who are sanctioned for non-compliance, for example, will be denied cash assistance through emergency services. Child welfare clients will be expected to make their own contacts, arrange their own transportation, and keep their own appointments without agency assistance. Clients who are removed from shelters as a result of their own poor behavior will be denied further shelter assistance by the county. While there are advantages to agency consistency, this approach denies clients the second chance that subsequent contact with the child welfare agency might otherwise provide.

Distortion in Agency Roles

Increased local discretion, which is the hallmark of the PRWORA, may result in inappropriate reordering of agency responsibilities, at the expense of the child welfare system. For example, one rural county in Virginia reported that foster care caseloads had significantly increased because the local judge decided that foster care was a reasonable alternative for youth who were truant from school. For working parents, especially those attempting to prove themselves in a new job, this presents a potential no-win situation. If a responsible parent goes to work, but then has less time to adequately supervise the children, the consequence may be foster care.

The Court has also been a factor in the District of Columbia where there is no separate Family Court and judges with no special training take turns overseeing child welfare cases. Some have mandated special schools and other costly treatment services for individual children, diverting funding that could otherwise be used to preserve or reunify families.

Staffing and Training

Lack of training has also been an issue among child welfare staff. In one jurisdiction in Maryland, an effort to contain costs in the face of increased foster care rolls resulted in the hiring of foster care workers on a contractual basis. Many lacked proper credentials or experience and received minimal training, resulting in high turnover, erratic screening, and poor judgments regarding children's safety, leading to exceptionally high foster care placement rates. More than twice as many cases of neglect and abuse ended up in foster care in this jurisdiction than elsewhere in the state. Additional placements resulting from welfare reform may further compound these problems.

Kinship Care

One of the ways that social service agencies have responded to children who have been removed from their homes is to put a priority on placing them with relatives. In Washington, D.C., for example, the new general receiver intends to use legal guardianship as the mechanism to secure stability for children in kinship care (E. Jones, personal communication, March 25, 1998). She also hopes to establish neighborhood centers where relatives/caretakers can come for help on an as-needed basis. She also plans to remove them from the foster care rolls. This will change the foster care data in the District significantly since about half of the current foster care cases are kinship care cases. She anticipates, as do her counterparts in Baltimore City, that as mothers reach the TANF time limits, many will look to relatives to care for their children when they can no longer afford to do so. To some advocates, this practice is viewed positively, and is seen as preferable to moving children out of their communities into foster homes in neighboring counties, a common practice at present. It is also viewed as preferable to placing African-American children in non-African-American homes. On the other hand, it will not honor the intent of welfare reform in making the biological mother more responsible or self-sufficient. It will also add to the problems associated with documenting the impact of welfare reform since, in many cases, mothers giving their children to relatives for care will not appear in any official statistics.

INNOVATIONS

The authors were impressed with several holistic approaches to promoting family well-being that were identified in conducting the study.

One suburban county in Maryland anticipated welfare reform in 1995, and began planning a "Family Investment" Program. The program puts the family's needs at the center of a comprehensive service package that includes employment assistance, job training, health care, and day care services, all at a single site. The county agency generated lists of prospective employers, but employers may be included in the job bank only if they agree to pay more than minimum wage. The agency has worked with clients to establish a transportation service (Wheels for Work) owned and operated by clients; contracted for services to respond to the special needs of women who are victims of domestic violence; and worked with the courts to mandate non-custodial parents to come to them to secure jobs, thus reducing the number of "deadbeat dads" in detention and increasing child support payments. The agency has also reduced foster care placements by having staff available 24 hours a day to resolve family conflicts and discourage placement.

The county also operates an "open-door" policy, so parents in crisis can use foster homes on a short term basis. Recidivism in this context is not considered a problem. For the alcoholic mother in recovery, a relapse is less traumatic and devastating for the children when they can contact the foster home and receive temporary care until mother resumes sobriety. While this might not be advisable in some cases (e.g., where there is concern about the potential danger of the substance abuser to the foster family), it has potential in others. In those cases, "success" should not be defined solely in terms of reliance on substitute care.

The Commonwealth of Virginia, through its Comprehensive Services Act, has mandated the use of Family Assessment Teams to meet the needs of high-risk children and families. These teams seem to be operating most successfully in the smaller counties, where there are fewer barriers to communication and collaboration both within and across agencies. One small rural county, for example, reports the successful use of teams comprising staff from the departments of Social Services, Court Services, Special Education, Mental Health, and Health. They meet with parents, as often as twice per month, to develop a comprehensive plan for the child and family, designed to prevent out-of-home care.

Richmond, Virginia, a large urban center, reports successful collaboration among its Department of Social Services, police department, juvenile courts, Health Department, and Department of Parks and Recreation. They share resources, including budget dollars, in support of shared priorities. They also integrate staff, as needed. For example, through a special initiative funded by the city, social workers are stationed in the police precinct so that intervention can begin at the first sign of need, particularly in cases of family violence. Welfare reform staff and staff from the Family Violence Prevention Program also work closely together. For example, when TANF recipients are screened, Family Violence staff are alerted to any domestic violence issues so that additional services can be provided. In some cases, where domestic violence threatens to make it impossible or unsafe for a TANF recipient to work, Family Violence has worked successfully with the welfare staff to arrange for a waiver or deferral of the welfare program's work requirement.

Several counties acknowledged that benefit terminations under welfare reform might lead to child welfare involvement, but are committed to preventing foster care as an outcome. One suburban county has begun to identify funding streams that can be pooled to assist families in this predicament, although they warn that the money will be easily depleted. One urban area is counting on its juvenile judges to put pressure on the county to provide services to vulnerable families, in order to avert the need for out-of-home placements. Other counties are counting on their legislature to step in and alter the stringent new requirements, rather than see children removed from home as a result of benefit reductions. For the most part, these responses remain untested.

RECOMMENDATIONS

On the basis of the information gathered, it is clear that child welfare agencies must begin to plan ahead for the possible repercussions of welfare reform. The following recommendations address the need for relevant, accurate data as well as the need for agency-based and service-based reforms.

Data Collection

It is important that data collection go beyond addressing reductions in the welfare rolls or even job placement rates, and begin addressing the well-being of low-income children. Foster care placements are one likely indicator of welfare's impact on children, yet separating out the impact of welfare reform from other variables affecting foster care will be a daunting task. After all, foster care rates can be influenced by a whole host of factors, including the idiosyncratic decisions of individual judges, trends in child abuse reporting, the relative success of family preservation efforts, consistency in implementing recent federal requirements for swifter termination of parental rights, reliance on kinship care and how it is reflected in foster care data, worker turnover and training, and the ability of staff to make sound placement decisions. Especially critical is the strength of the economy and its impact on family poverty. Research efforts attempting to link welfare reform to changes in foster care rolls will have to take each of these variables into account.

Data collection efforts in this area will also need to address not only those who reach the time limit and are forced off the rolls, but also those who lose benefits through being sanctioned, those who leave the rolls voluntarily (for example, substance abusers and those with mental or physical disabilities who are unwilling or unable to follow through with program requirements), those who fail to qualify for benefits (for example, some foreign born applicants), and those who are discouraged from applying in the first place. One large Virginia county notes that, while its welfare rolls are at an all-time low, its inquiries are at an all-time high, suggesting that there are families in need who are not availing themselves of cash when they learn of the new strings attached. A substantially increased demand for community services lends credibility to this conclusion.

While our welfare policy may attempt to distinguish between those who do and do not deserve to receive benefits, it is important that our data make no such judgments and that we conscientiously track *all* low-income children who are in any way affected by the new welfare rules.

It is also important that data collection be long-term and nationwide, and that it examine jurisdictions with both strong and weak economies. Any research on children in foster care must include the growing number of children in kinship care. Likewise, some children whose families are impacted by welfare reform might have subsequent contact with systems other than child welfare–most notably mental health or juvenile justice. The experiences of these children, too, must be reflected in any research on the effects of welfare reform.

Agency Reform

Our findings suggest that child welfare agencies are already behind the curve in planning for the possible impact of welfare reform. Some repercussions are inevitable, and the potential for a major upheaval is real. With child welfare personnel and resources already strained to the limit in many agencies, few are well-positioned to deal constructively with the possible influx of needy families.

Child welfare agencies should begin to plan ahead NOW. A stable workforce of qualified staff is crucial to making sound assessments and placement decisions. Child welfare staff should be educated about the new welfare law, its limits, its opportunities, and its possible consequences for child welfare practice. Welfare program staff should be trained in assessment so that TANF families can be supported by appropriate services, forestalling later involvement with the child welfare system. New working relationships should be explored and negotiated within and between child welfare and welfare reform staff, encouraging collaboration around client families. Finally, all judges who preside over family court cases should be adequately prepared to deal knowledgeably and responsibly with abuse, neglect, termination, and placement decisions.

Service Availability

With the current emphasis on moving TANF recipients into jobs, it is critical that we not forget the importance of social support services in successfully lifting families out of poverty. After all, "the question of how work improves the well-being of the poor will . . . be tied up with what other types of public and private assistance are available to working low-income women" (Blank, 1997, p. 174).

Programs for substance-abusing women (including inpatient and residential treatment) are critical, given the degree to which drug addiction can interfere with both the ability to keep a job and the ability to parent one's children.

Safe, affordable child care is another priority. Without it, parents are placed in the untenable position of having to choose between working (with the promise of "self-sufficiency") and ensuring that their children are safe and supervised. There is an especially pressing need for infant care, for specialized child care for children with special needs, and for subsidized care for older children who are too often left alone. Table 1 summarizes our recommendations.

It is important to remember that moving TANF recipients into jobs is a starting point, not the ultimate goal. Too often, clients successfully take jobs only to find themselves without the safety net of cash assistance *and* without enough income to support their families. It would be ironic for our society to embrace a work ethic that results in the impoverishment of our children.

TABLE 1

RECOMMENDATIONS TO STATES
PERFORM DATA COLLECTION THAT NOTES ANY IMPACT PRWORA HAS ON CHILDREN • Account for the wide variety of direct and indirect factors that impact on child welfare involvement • Collect nationwide and long-term data across economic conditions • Recognize overlap effects among child serving and welfare agencies **PLAN AHEAD FOR REPERCUSSIONS IN CHILD WELFARE** • Increase retention of qualified staff • Increase communication among social service staff within and across agencies • Cross train judges, income support, and child welfare staff **INCREASE SERVICE AVAILABILITY** • Safe and affordable child care • Transportation in remote areas • Use of flexible foster care option • Drug treatment services

Salaries, or a combination of salaries and public assistance, must be sufficient to allow those who work to earn a living wage, one that meets actual day-to-day expenses and allows for the accumulation of savings. Savings are especially important should our economy not maintain its current strength. Economic change could be a major factor in the success or failure of welfare reform.

CONCLUSION

We run the risk of viewing welfare reform too narrowly. It is not simply about whether the welfare rolls are getting smaller; it is not simply about how much money we spend on cash assistance, or who deserves help, or how to discourage dependence on government. Nor is it simply about moving adults into jobs. It is first and foremost about the well-being of children. They should, after all, be the primary beneficiaries of our welfare policies.

Keeping the focus on the well-being of children requires that our research on the impact of welfare reform go beyond tracking how many TANF recipients move into jobs and how many exhaust their benefits; it must commit itself to determining what impact, if any, the new welfare rules have on the children in all of these families. The tightening of requirements for TANF recipients under the Personal Responsibility and Work Opportunity Reconciliation Act will inevitably leave some families with fewer resources. What will be the consequences? To answer this question responsibly, we will have to look not just to the welfare system, but to the child welfare system, the schools, the juvenile justice system, the mental health system, and all systems that serve children in need.

The availability of information about the impact of welfare reform on child welfare is limited, since relatively little time has elapsed since new welfare programs were put into place. There is reason to believe that the reduced financial resources available to some families may lead to subsequent contacts with various child-serving systems–chief among them, child welfare. If so, it is important for those agencies to ready themselves, and carve out for themselves a role which can be positive and constructive in the lives of these families. For those clients who are unsuccessful in achieving "self-sufficiency" under welfare reform, later contact with another agency should serve not as a punishment, but as a second chance in the struggle to ensure the well-being of their children.

REFERENCES

Baratz, M. & White, S. (1996). Childfare: A new direction for welfare reform. *Urban Studies*, *33*, 1935-1944.

Blank, R.M. (1997). Policy watch: The 1996 welfare reform. *Journal of Economic Perspectives*, *11* (1), 169-177.

Brown, M. (1998, April 16). Bracing to embrace the poor. *The Burke Times*, p. A11.

Burnam, A. & Melamid, E. (1998). Child protection and welfare reform. http://www.rand.org/publications/CF/CF123.

Child Welfare League of America (1997, Aug. 7). *CWLA welfare reform and child welfare summary*, Washington, DC: Author.

Children's Defense Fund (1998). *The state of America's children.* Washington, D.C.

Collins, A. & Aber, J.L. (1998). How welfare reform can help or hurt children. *Children and Welfare Reform: Issue Brief 1.* New York: National Center for Children in Poverty.

Courtney, M. (1995). The foster care crisis and welfare reform. *Public Welfare, 53* (3), 27-40.

Courtney, M. (1997). Child welfare in the context of welfare reform. In S. Kamerman & A. Kahn (Eds.), *Child Welfare in the Context of Welfare Reform* (Report V) (pp. 1-35). New York: Cross-National Studies Research Program, Columbia University School of Social Work.

Geen, R. & Waters, S. (1997, Nov.). The Impact of welfare reform on child welfare financing. *New Federalism: Issues and Options for States* (Number A-16). Washington, DC: The Urban Institute. http://newfederalism.urban.org/html/anf16.html.

Hardin, M. (1997). Sizing up the welfare act's impact on child protection. *Clearinghouse Review, 30*, 1061-1068.

Knitzer, J. & Bernard, S. (1998). The new welfare law and vulnerable families: Implications for child welfare/child protection systems. *Children and Welfare Reform: Issue Brief 3.* New York: National Center for Children in Poverty.

Pavetti, L., Olson, K., Nightingale, D., Duke, A., & Isaacs, J. (1997). *Welfare-to-work options for families facing personal and family challenges: Rationale and program strategies*. Washington, D.C.: Urban Institute.

Videka-Sherman, L. & Viggiani, P. (1996). The impact of federal policy changes on children: Research needs for the future. *Social Work, 41*, 594-600.

Vobejda, B. & Havemann, J. (1998, April 13). States' welfare data in disarray. *The Washington Post*, pp. A1, A7.

Delinquency Prevention in Poor and At-Risk African-American Youth: A Social Work Practice Innovation

Michael Forster
Timothy Rehner

SUMMARY. Juvenile delinquency is a major social issue today which threatens to become more acute with anticipated demographic shifts and reductions in public support for the poor. Effective strategies for the prevention and reduction of delinquency among poor and at-risk youth are much needed. The Family Network Partnership is a small community-based delinquency prevention program in Hattiesburg, Mississippi. The program joins the city housing authority, the community policing team, the youth court, and the local state university in efforts to address delinquency in a local public housing project. The program uses three primary strategies: (1) intervention with youth already involved with the juvenile justice system; (2) skill-building among youth prior to court involvement; and (3) community capacity building. This paper describes the Partnership's background, principles and program, and outcomes to date. With qualification, the Partnership is offered as a model for replication in similar communities. *[Article copies available for a fee from The Haworth Document Delivery Service: 1-800-342-9678. E-mail address: getinfo@haworthpressinc.com <Website: http://www.haworthpressinc.com>]*

KEYWORDS. Delinquency prevention, delinquency reduction, at-risk youth, poor youth, community building

Juvenile delinquency is a major social problem with recognized links to poverty and related indicators as inner-city residence, substandard schooling,

---

Michael Forster, PhD, and Timothy Rehner, PhD, are Assistant Professors of Social Work, The University of Southern Mississippi.

[Haworth co-indexing entry note]: "Delinquency Prevention in Poor and At-Risk African-American Youth: A Social Work Practice Innovation." Forster, Michael, and Timothy Rehner. Co-published simultaneously in *Social Thought* (The Haworth Pastoral Press, an imprint of The Haworth Press, Inc.) Vol. 19, No. 2, 1999, pp. 37-52; and: *Raising Our Children Out of Poverty* (ed: John J. Stretch et al.) The Haworth Pastoral Press, an imprint of The Haworth Press, Inc., 1999, pp. 37-52. Single or multiple copies of this article are available for a fee from The Haworth Document Delivery Service [1-800-342-9678, 9:00 a.m. - 5:00 p.m. (EST). E-mail address: getinfo@haworthpressinc.com].

inadequate health care, and single-parent, female-headed homes. Rates of violent crime by juveniles, after remaining stable for a decade, leapt dramatically from 1988 to 1994 (Mulvey, Arthur & Reppucci, 1997). At the moment rates of crime are again declining overall, probably at least in part due to a declining proportion of teenagers in the population. As continuing waves of "baby boomer" offspring come into adolescence, however, there is danger that juvenile delinquency will again surge.

The danger is increased by the growing numbers of poor children and youth growing up homeless, in single-parent, "latchkey" home situations, and in crime-ridden neighborhoods. Presently over one-quarter of America's children live in poverty, with estimates running as high as one-third by the end of the decade (O'Donnell et al., 1997). In Mississippi, poverty rates for children already exceed 33% and are expected to grow in the wake of welfare reform efforts (Borom, 1998). At the same time, funding for social programs that might cushion the impact of poverty has decreased significantly as conservative social philosophy has moved into political ascendancy. Effective strategies for the prevention and reduction of juvenile delinquency are, therefore, much needed.

This paper concerns the Family Network Partnership project (FNP), a small community-based delinquency prevention program directed by the authors, faculty members at The University of Southern Mississippi (USM) School of Social Work in Hattiesburg, Mississippi. Now in its third year of operation, FNP's focus is on youth and families residing in a 175-unit Hattiesburg public housing project and the immediately surrounding community. The vast majority of residents are poor, and the remainder live near the poverty line, usually one payroll, disability or social security check away from crisis. Data indicate community youth at-risk for poor school performance, dropping out before finishing high school, involvement with the juvenile justice system, high dependence on social welfare services, and inconsistent, low-wage employment (City of Hattiesburg, 1993).

The FNP lives in the spirit of professional social work's long tradition of community-based practice and applied research. While the Partnership learns and grows daily, its aim is not so much new knowledge acquisition per se as it is the application of what we already have good reason to believe "works" to address youth, family, and community problems associated with chronic poverty and dependence.

This paper will in turn describe the FNP's background, its principles of operation, the main lines of its program and organizational structure, and the preparation of students for work in the program. Outcomes and implications of the program to date are briefly addressed, as are the major challenges currently faced. With qualification, the FNP experience is offered as a model for replication in similar poor communities.

BACKGROUND

History and Purpose

The FNP is proof that ideas have consequences. The genesis of the Partnership was a late 1994 colloquium event, "Youth Violence and the Failures of Community," produced by The University of Southern Mississippi School of Social Work. An analysis by the lead author (Forster, 1994) located the principal source of youth violence in the decay of community institutions–schools, churches, local businesses, voluntary civic organizations, government and other public agencies–in their capacity to support families in their socializing tasks. Poverty per se was not identified as a problem. However, communities of concentrated poverty were found to be at greatest risk of youth problems because they were, typically, bereft of adequate community support resources.

Participants in the colloquium included the Hattiesburg police chief and the county youth court judge responsible for handling all local delinquency cases. Ideas that emerged from the colloquium struck a responsive chord, and in a subsequent meeting, the authors were challenged to develop a social work response to the growing problem of youth crime in Hattiesburg's poorest communities.

The authors spent most of 1995 forming relationships with community players, reviewing relevant literature, discussing various approaches, and seeking financial and in-kind support for an intervention effort. Discussions involved the youth court, the police (who had just months before launched a community policing effort in the city's high crime districts), the city's recreation and planning departments, the public child welfare and health agencies, a smattering of public school and community organizations (churches, boys' and girls' clubs), and community residents themselves.

Through an inclusive process of dialogue, we built consensus in favor of a project that would attempt to:

1. Reduce the penetration of troubled youth into the juvenile justice system.
2. Strengthen the key socialization institutions–family and community–in order to improve general well-being and to prevent delinquency among poor and at-risk youth.
3. Improve key public systems performance on behalf of poor children and families through networking and collaboration.
4. Advance social justice and racial equality in communities historically characterized by pervasive discrimination and injustice.

Buoyed by extensive moral support and promises of limited logistical assistance (but no funding), we launched the Partnership in spring of 1996 as an unfunded project of the School of Social Work. The authors served as directors, and our workers were social work student interns in the bachelor's and master's degree programs. The public schools, and later the housing authority, contributed office space. The police set up a city phone line and answering machine, the recreation department donated office furniture. The youth court provided access to the detention center and set up a reliable screening and referral system.

With this minimal infrastructure in place, in the fall of 1996 the authors successfully secured approximately $50,000 in funding from the Mississippi Department of Public Safety, charged with dispensing federal Office of Juvenile Justice and Delinquency Prevention. This money permitted hiring the first (and only) full-time employee of the Partnership, a coordinator holding the MSW degree. The coordinator serves as the organizational linchpin of the Partnership. While the directors provide oversight and retain signature authority on the grant, the coordinator manages all day-to-day operations, and, in the capacity of field instructor for the School of Social Work, directs the activities of students.

The Community

The FNP is located within the Robertson Place Apartments, a 140-unit public housing project on Hattiesburg's east side. Robertson and the immediately surrounding community is the focus of FNP activity, with more than 90% of services provided to residents of this area. The community is characterized by ethnic homogeneity, poverty, high rates of crime, and limited opportunities for youth to engage in positive socialization activities.

The east side is the oldest section of Hattiesburg (population, approximately 70,000). Over the years, most middle and upper income residents, along with most whites, have followed the growth trail west. Thus while Hattiesburg's overall racial composition is about 68% white and 32% black, the district surrounding Robertson Place is 95% black. The population of Robertson Place itself is 100% black.

The overwhelming majority of residents in the FNP's focal community are poor. The mean annual income of Robertson Place residents in 1997 was $5,800. Among those who worked, the mean hourly wage was $5.80. While mean incomes in the surrounding district are somewhat higher, census data suggest that over 60% of families living in the area fall below the poverty line, approximately twice the rate of poverty in Mississippi, poorest state in the nation, as a whole. Approximately 40% of households in the area are headed by single women. Education levels of area residents are low, with less than a majority completing high school. Employment opportunities of any type not requiring private transportation are scarce; living wage jobs are virtually non-existent in the area.

Key Players

While the Partnership continually extends its network of relationships, key participants are, in addition to the School of Social Work, the Hattiesburg Police Department (in particular, the "Neighborhood Enhancement Team"–N.E.T.–the community policing unit), the Forrest County Youth Court, the Hattiesburg Housing Authority, the community residents' association, and the Department of Therapeutic Recreation at the University of Southern Mississippi. Other, more occasional participants include the public schools, the public health, mental health and child welfare agencies, local churches, and various individual faculty within the university.

PROGRAM AND PRINCIPLES

From the vast ocean of literature pertinent to delinquency, we have drawn primarily upon five broadly conceptualized currents–those related to social learning theory and psychoeducationally oriented youth work; ecologically oriented casework and service systems integration; family support and family-centered intervention; community building; and strength-based, solution-focused, short-term intervention. Rather than attempt the formidable task of a separate literature review, we identify below the major strategies and underlying principles that have shaped our project design and implementation choices, referencing a representative selection of literature as we go.

Program Strategies

The Family Network Partnership uses three general strategies to reduce and prevent juvenile crime in Robertson Place and the immediately surrounding community.

The first strategy is early intervention with youth already involved with the county youth court. Without intervention, a majority of juvenile first offenders are likely to commit a second offense (Quinn, Bell, & Ward, 1997). Prevention and early intervention strategies, not surprisingly, figure prominently into the literature on delinquency related behaviors. Thus advocates such as Edelman (1994) and Schorr (1989) point to the high cost–not only in terms of delinquency but myriad other interlocking pathologies–of widespread but preventable social neglect of at-risk children. Treatment strategists addressing a wide range of delinquency related problems–such as conduct and oppositional defiant disorders (Horne & Sayger, 1990), substance abuse (Rhodes & Jason, 1988), and sex offending (Gray & Pithers, 1993)–recommend early assessment and intervention for best rehabilitative success.

Referrals of first- and second-time offenders from the target community are made to FNP by the youth court. Following an ecological assessment taking into account individual, family and systemic factors, Partnership staff look to engage the youth's family and other relevant and influential community agents–school teachers, police, employers, health and mental health providers, churches and neighborhood organizations–to address immediate needs and improve coping capacities. Ecological approaches of this type have a proven track record with troubled youth (see, e.g., Hobbs, 1982; Whittaker, 1980) dating back more than twenty years, and have emerged as a cornerstone of revised thinking about effective intervention.

Time-limited individualized case plans are used to organize and evaluate planned intervention. The basic methodology is social casework (Compton & Galaway, 1994) informed by Partnership principles (see below). The range of possible interventions is extensive and inclusive, from direct counseling and skill instruction to some form of systems advocacy and referral for one or another type of specialized service(s) (see case vignette below). In cases where the risk of reoffense is considered especially high, involvement of the community policing team is a prominent feature of case plans. A variety of studies (e.g., Brewer et al., 1995; Skogan & Wycoff, 1986) have confirmed the common sense perception that a sustained high level of police and court involvement with youth is a significant deterrent of delinquent behavior.

The Partnership's second strategy is to develop positive skills and capacities *before* they engage in delinquent behaviors. Competency deficits of various types, including academic, social skill, and anger management deficiencies, constitute significant risk factors for delinquency (Goldstein & Glick, 1987; Strayhorn, 1988; Forster & McCarthy, 1995). Deliberate cultivation of competencies, conversely, can promote resilience (Anthony & Cohler, 1987), while inhibiting the development of delinquent behaviors. Examining social learning approaches, researchers such as Goldstein (1988) and Forman (1993) have demonstrated the effectiveness of time-limited programs in teaching skill-deficient youth competencies ranging from problem-solving to stress management and cooperation. In a similar vein, Durkin, Forster, and Linton (1989; Forster, Linton, & Durkin, 1987) have indicated the use of a competency perspective to ground more extended residential and community-based programs for high-risk youth.

FNP builds competencies in the community's young people through tutoring, recreational activities, cultural events, a gardening project, community service opportunities, and peer-oriented skill development (for teens). As Vorrath and Brendtro (1985) have indicated, the power of the peer group can be effectively tapped to build a culture of positive values and learning among high-risk youth. In addition, the Partnership operates a lending library of children's books, runs a popular "token store" which provides earned rewards for youth who demonstrate pro-social behaviors, and maintains a schedule of "drop-in" hours at the office.

The Partnership's third strategy is to reduce environmental risk factors through community capacity building. Robertson Place is a relatively isolated community characterized by limited internal "youth friendly" resources–recreational, cultural, spiritual, age-appropriate work, community service, and the like. The absence of such community resources is associated with high risk for delinquency (Hawkins, Catalano & Brewer, 1995); their presence, conversely, contributes to the resiliency of at-risk youth (Carnegie Council, 1991; Thornberry, Huizinga & Loeber, 1995). Moreover, numerous financial, transportation and social barriers severely restrict the ability of youth and families to access resources external to the immediate community. Perhaps worst of all, many if not most residents feel powerless to effect substantial change in their life circumstances.

The Partnership addresses these issues through a range of resident/community empowerment activities. In the first place, the agency itself has literally "joined" the community. Its office adjoins the apartments' community center, and residents are encouraged to "drop in" for casual visits. FNP staff are visible and widely known in the community. There is a possibility that in the near future a staff member will take up personal residence in the community. Second, we engage the community in program development. We have based all programs for youth on needs assessments conducted with residents, and residents have been involved in planning these programs. Some residents volunteer in the programs, working alongside FNP staff. We collaborate with indigenous community agents, such as local churches, to enhance their own services and opportunities for families and youth in order to make the community more "youth friendly." Third, we encourage residents in taking concrete steps to take more control over their lives. We offer consultation and training to parents on working with their children, and on advocating for their own interests with public service providers. We participate in the planning and execution of community residents' meetings. We have spearheaded one voter registration drive and intend more in the future.

Principles

These general strategies rest upon a number of more-or-less evident premises. Most notable are the following:

Social work should join the community. Central to the at-risk condition of many youth in the Robertson Place neighborhood is the relative weakness of community institutions to carry out the function of socializing young people. Conversely, the needs of at-risk youth will be addressed to the extent that the entire community is strengthened and empowered to mobilize its own resources in the tasks of socialization. The social work tradition, of course, runs deep in its emphasis on community organization, development and empowerment. Long before the current surge of interest in "local control" approaches to social issues, social workers have sought to "partner" with local forces (Ehrenreich, 1985; Kahn, 1995). The FNP attempts to return social work to its community-based, and justice-oriented roots in this regard (Specht & Courtney, 1994), demonstrating how it works "in public" (Fisher & Karger, 1997).

Social work should partner with police. From the standpoint of preventing youth penetration of the juvenile justice system, police/social worker collaboration in particular is critical. The community policing approach seems overall sound, and is gathering kudos from every quarter (Lacayo, 1996; Thurman, 1995). Fay (1998), both a psychologist and a police officer, finds that "good police work resembles good therapy." By itself, however, community policing is insufficient to address the needs of at-risk youth effectively. In the final analysis community police officers are agents of law enforcement, not social workers. Expecting officers to employ social work helping methodology would be impractical and cause blurring of important role distinctions. (As an N.E.T. officer said, "When push comes to shove, my job is to get the bad guys off the street.") On the other hand, the practicality of police/social work collaboration has been well-established (Treger, 1989). In an atmosphere of cooperation and joint consultation, and with proper training, police/social work teams can dramatically enhance a community's response to crime and delinquency (Treger, 1995). Using social workers to enhance the N.E.T. project is, therefore, an extension of an existing record of success. In a similar way, the N.E.T. is often a vital element in individual case plans, especially with more difficult, delinquency-prone youth.

Systems collaboration and integration is pivotal. Beyond the police-social work bond, broader system integration is imperative to addressing the needs of at-risk youth effectively. All the major systems that impact these young people and their families–welfare, education, recreation, health and mental health, as well as the police and courts–must be "on the same page" in efforts to craft useful and cost effective intervention strategies. The need for improved collaboration is an outstanding theme of the nascent "family support" movement, which we believe has much to offer to community-based efforts at delinquency prevention (see especially Kagan & Weissbourd, 1994). Often the main reason for ineffective work with disturbed and delinquent young people is not the intractability of their problems but rather that our fragmented systems of juvenile justice, child welfare, and mental health simply allow youth to "fall through the cracks" (see, e.g., Combrinck-Graham, 1990).

Even in so-called resource deprived communities, duplication of services and program overlap by various independent agencies is not uncommon

(U.S. General Accounting Office, 1996). More common, however, are significant gaps in services, especially in the provision of concrete family support services, and services offered at times and locations convenient for recipients and responsive to recipient input and feedback (Massinga, 1994). These issues will likely only be addressed in poor communities through improved provider collaboration, integration of services, and reconceptualization of worker roles (Goetz & Peck, 1994; Mulroy, 1997).

Families remain central to success. At-risk youth rarely present problems outside a family context. A family centered approach to helping, featuring attention to issues of the family ecology, family developmental stage, and parental competence (Pecora, Whitakker and Maluccio, 1992), is, we believe, more likely to bear fruit than approaches that focus more-or-less exclusive attention on individual delinquents or even peer groups. FNP workers draw upon the extensive practice literature on effective work with multi-problem families and families with delinquent children (see, for example, Schaefer, Briesmeister & Fitton, 1984). To the greatest extent possible, resources of the family system (including extended family and community resources) of the at-risk youth should be identified, mobilized and engaged (Clark, 1994; Kagan & Schlosberg, 1989).

Rapid, significant change is possible. While the reality of family dysfunction should not be ignored or denied, the Partnership believes that "strength-based," "solution-focused" work with families and troubled youth will yield better results, faster, than traditional psychodynamic, "pathologizing" approaches (Kaplan and Girard, 1994). This helping perspective assumes that: (a) all individuals and families have both internal and external strengths and resources that can be built upon to address deficits and problems most effectively; and (b) individuals and systems can often achieve practical solutions without paying extended attention to the "roots" of their difficulties (O'Hanlon & Weiner-Davis, 1989). This premise helps to ground the brief and frequently intermittent style of intervention that workers employ with youth and families. Because FNP is literally an ever-present part of the community, families can utilize services on an episodic basis, briefly but without ever losing contact with the agency; Kreilkamp (1989) described a similar model in use with a community health maintenance organization in Cambridge, Massachusetts. The solution-focused orientation incorporates, further, a wide range of specific "constructivist" (Foyt, 1996) and related techniques. We have been especially influenced by the work of Selekman (1996) with youth, and Berg (1994) with families.

Illustrative Case Vignette

The Brown case illustrates FNP's non-traditional service approach. Already known to most local service providers, the Brown family was referred to FNP because 11-year-old Tommy was caught selling stolen beer in the neighborhood. A rapid assessment revealed that the single parent, Pam, had two younger children, was eight months pregnant with her fourth child, and faced two outstanding bench warrants for arrest on drug charges. The immediate living situation was desperate–little food in the house, utilities turned off, and the landlord threatening eviction.

Partnership workers affirmed Pam's goal to hold her family together, and to take concrete steps to resolve her many issues. Through meetings and negotiations with key system players–family members, courts, police, child protection services, health and mental health care providers, and other community agencies–FNP helped Pam cobble together a realistic plan for herself and her kids. She pre-registered with a maternity unit and entered a drug treatment program with her youngest child. The other children were voluntarily placed with relatives. Workers enlisted local agencies in getting the utilities turned on and postponing possible eviction.

The case is on-going. Tommy is in counseling, and Pam will be offered in-home services when she completes in-patient treatment. Because FNP workers moved quickly and flexibly in a family-centered way, delinquency was averted, a family was sustained, and a community's capacity to respond to people in crisis was strengthened.

WORKER PREPARATION

Operating successfully in a community-based program housed within an impoverished public housing project requires preparation somewhat different than the norm in social work education today. Acknowledging that the following is something of a caricature, we would contend that normative social work education prepares students to: focus on client pathology; operate in an office-bound context; specialize their problem-solving practice; play well-defined agency roles; distinguish these roles sharply from those of other professions; and maintain a keen sense of their own professional posture.

Preparation of FNP student/workers, by contrast, moves in the opposite direction on each of the above points. Workers are trained to avoid pathologizing labeling in favor of "solution talk" with clients. They are not office-bound, but function as "life space" practitioners who view the entire community, the natural ecology of the children and families, as their field of activity. Workers do not specialize, but approach problems-to-be-solved in the mode of generalists prepared to act flexibly, comprehensively, and creatively to move plans along. Roles are, as a result, multiple and fluid, and frequently overlap with those usually associated with other professional or para-professionals, such as therapeutic recreation and child care/youth development workers. Far from professional posturing, workers strive to be "good neighbors" to community members, erasing as much of the social distance between residents and themselves as possible.

In order to assist students preparing for FNP work, the directors have devised a twenty-hour orientation training as prerequisite to the field experience. The curriculum for this training draws heavily from the European "social pedagogy" (Linton, 1971; Beker & Barnes, 1990) and American "re-educational" (Hobbs, 1982) approaches to working with difficult youth. These approaches emphasize interventive activity in the total life space of clients. Students are oriented to the community itself, FNP principles, and a variety of fundamental skills, including the rudiments of solution-focused work, behavior modification, activity management, life-space interviewing and responding to aggressive behavior (Forster and Rehner, 1997).

OUTCOMES AND IMPLICATIONS

Available data suggest that the FNP is on track toward meeting its primary goals of (1) reducing the penetration of troubled youth into the juvenile justice system; (2) strengthening the capacity of families and the community to prevent delinquency; (3) improving collaboration among public service providers; and (4) advancing social justice.

Unfortunately, at this point hard data on outcomes are limited and relate principally to the goal of reducing system penetration. Police records indicate a dramatic 25% drop in juvenile crime in the target community between 1996 and 1997. While the Partnership would gladly take credit for this impressive development, the decline in local crime parallels a general decline in both juvenile and adult crime in the city as a whole. Perhaps more significant are preliminary figures from the youth court suggesting that less than 20% of youth referred to the Partnership and subsequently worked with have committed additional offenses within the twelve-month period following referral. While this rate of recidivism appears significantly below the prevailing norm, no appropriate comparison group has yet been examined to validiate this impression.

Data collection is underway regarding the goal of strengthening family and community capacity. Baseline data on family functioning in areas of communication style, parenting/discipline methods, access and utilization of resources, and patterns of coping (cf. Kagan & Schlosberg, 1989) are collected routinely for families participating in case plans. A baseline of community self-perception of capacity has been determined in the context of a larger needs assessment. It remains, however, to aggregate family outcomes data and to reassess the perception of community capacity after a sufficient period of time.

More abundant soft data are encouraging. Feedback on FNP activity from major partners–housing authority, police department, and youth court–is unequivocally positive, the consensus being that the Partnership is "making a difference" with individual youth and families, and with the community as a whole. The program has gained some noted recognition from authorities, including a recent citation as one of three programs that has put Hattiesburg in the running for a national award as a "most livable city" (McCann, April 22, 1998).

Acceptance of the Partnership in the Robertson Place community has steadily grown among both youth and adult residents. Early expectations that the program (like some previous university-based efforts) would leave the community after a short time have given way to treatment of FNP staff as reliable "neighbors."

Improvement of public systems performance is an elusive outcome, difficult to measure empirically. Early indications are encouraging, however. Responsiveness to youth and family needs has unquestionably been enhanced through FNP advocacy. In addition to the youth court, police and housing authority, the Partnership has successfully engaged the public child welfare agency, the public and private mental health systems, and the public schools. At the schools' invitation, FNP is currently exploring the feasibility of running positive peer culture groups (Vorrath & Brendtro, 1985) with at-risk youth referred by school personnel. Substantive collaborative ventures are still in their infancy, however.

Social justice is, of course, a long-term project, which will be measured, in part, by the breaking down of the community's insularity, the increased engagement of a widening circle of external "partners" with community residents in ways that strengthen the community and make headway against poverty, and diminished stereotyping of the residents, the community, and public housing. Though early, the prospects for significant gains along these dimensions are good. In addition to the public and private partnership ties already noted, promising connections have been made with local and state organizations espousing strong social justice missions, including churches and Mississippi Families for Kids, an advocacy organization based in the state capital of Jackson. The University of Southern Mississippi stands in a very strong position in the Hattiesburg community. Its activities garner significant media attention, permitting FNP leaders to regularly spotlight its social justice aims.

CONCLUSION

The Family Network Partnership represents, we believe, a replicable model of cost-effective community-based social work. Drawing upon the profession's rich tradition of community-based practice, utilizing student interns extensively, and leveraging the prestige of the university into collaborative arrangements with public and private community agents, a university school of social work is ideally positioned to provide leadership to partnerships designed to address juvenile delinquency in poor communities. With minimal financial resources, schools, through the use of student interns and faculty with service and research interests, can sustain a vital level of direct intervention and community strengthening services.

Significant challenges remain, of course. An information system useful for evaluation and research purposes has yet to be developed. Despite overall success, collaboration with the key partners–youth court, police, housing authority, neighborhood association–remains difficult (cf. Mulroy, 1997) and administratively time-consuming, with issues of "turf," priorities for action, control of resources, and communication arising at nearly every turn. Heavy student placement with the FNP has identified, further, important curriculum gaps. Among other things, we have discovered students' preparation for assessment and case planning with poor African-American youth and families to be inadequate. Juvenile delinquency and content related to youth development generally is, further, barely addressed in the curriculum (cf. Sutphen, 1997). With some students, too, race and class stereotyping has been a salient issue. Finally, stability and limitation of funding is a priority concern. The current funding stream is time-limited, with perhaps another eighteen months of funding at the current level, and as yet no replacement dollars have been identified. One can make do with very little, indeed, but one must have at least something on a sustained basis to make do at all.

REFERENCES

Anthony, E. & Cohler, B. (Eds.) (1987). *The invulnerable child.* New York: Guilford Press.

Beker, J. & Barnes, F. (1990). The educateur returns to America: Approaching the development of professional child and youth care cross-culturally through ILEX. *Child and Youth Care Quarterly, 19,* 3: 161-175.

Berg, I.S. (1994). *Family-based services: A solution-focused approach.* W.W. Norton.

Borom, G. (1998). *Their future is in our hands: Recommendations for the eradication of child poverty in Mississippi.* Biloxi, MS: Congregations for Children/ Moore Community House.

Brewer, D.D., Hawkins, J.D., Catalan, R.F., & Neckerman, H.J. (1995). Preventing serious, violent, and chronic juvenile offending: A review of evaluations of selected strategies in childhood, adolescence, and the community. In J.C. Howell, B. Krisberg, J. Hawkins, & J. Wilson (Eds.), *Serious, violent, & chronic juvenile offender: A sourcebook.* (pp. 61-141). Sage Publications.

Bynum, J. & Thompson, W. (1989). *Juvenile delinquency: A sociological approach.* Boston: Allyn & Bacon.

Carnegie Council on Adolescent Development. (1991). *A matter of time: Risk and opportunity in the nonschool hours.* New York: Carnegie Corporation of New York.

City of Hattiesburg (1993, October 12). *City of Hattiesburg police hiring supplement program.* (Funding proposal submitted to the U.S. Dept. of Justice, Washington, DC). Hattiesburg, Mississippi.

Clark, M. (1996). Brief solution-focused work: A strengths-based method for juvenile justice practice. *Juvenile and Family Court Journal*, 47, 1: 57-65.

Combrinck-Graham, L. (1990). *Giant steps: Therapeutic innovations in child mental health.* Basic Books.

Compton, B. & Galaway, B. (1994). *Social work processes.* Pacific Grove, CA: Brooks/Cole.

Durkin, R., Forster, M. & Linton, T. (1989). The Sage Hill program for competency promotion. In E. A. Balcerzak, (Ed.), *Group care of children: Transitions toward the year 2000.* (pp. 297-313). Washington, DC: Child Welfare League of America.

Edelman, M. (1994). Introduction. In Children's Defense Fund, *Wasting America's future.* (pp. xv-xxix). Boston: Beacon Press.

Ehrenreich, J. (1985). *The altruistic imagination: A history of social work and social policy in the United States.* Cornell University Press.

Fay, J. (1998). Therapists in blue. *Family Therapy Networker.* May/June, pp. 59-63, 67.

Fisher, R. & Karger, H. (1997). *Social work and community in a private world: Getting out in public.* Longman.

Forman, S.G. (1993). *Coping skills interventions for children and adolescents.* San Francisco: Jossey-Bass.

Forster, M., Linton, T.E., & Durkin, R. (1987). The promotion of competence in U.S. residential care: A model. *Residential Treatment for Children & Youth*, 5, 2, pp. 95-112.

Forster, M. (1994). Youth violence and the failures of community. *School of Social Work Colloquium Series.* Hattiesburg, MS: The University of Southern Mississippi School of Social Work.

Forster, M. & Rehner, T. (1997). *The Family Network Partnership: Preparing social work interns for community-based practice.* Paper presented at the 1997 annual meeting of the Alabama-Mississippi Social Work Education Conference. Mississippi State University, October 2-4, 1997.

Forster, M. & McCarthy, K. (1995). The aggression treatment project. *Contributions to Residential Treatment.* Alexandria, VA: American Association of Children's Residential Centers.

Foyt, M.F. (Ed.). (1996). *Constructivist therapies 2.* Guilford Press.

Goetz, K. & Peck, S. (Eds.). (1994). *The basics of family support: A guide for state planners.* Chicago: Family Resource Coalition.

Goldstein, A. & Glick, B. (1987). *Aggression replacement training.* Champaign, IL: Research Press.

Goldstein, A. (1988). *The prepare curriculum.* Champaign, Illinois: Research Press.

Gray, A.S. & Pithers, W.D. (1993). Relapse prevention with sexually aggressive adolescents and children: Expanding treatment and supervision. In H.E. Barbaree,

W.L. Marshall, & S.M. Hudson (Eds.), *The juvenile sex offender.* (pp. 289-319). Guilford Press.

Hawkins, J., Catalano, R., & Brewer, D. (1995). Preventing serious, violent, and chronic juvenile offending. In J.C. Howell, B. Krisberg, J. Hawkins, & J. Wilson, (Eds.), *Serious, violent, & chronic juvenile offender: A sourcebook.* (pp. 47-60). Sage Publications.

Hobbs, N. (1982). *The troubled and troubling child.* San Francisco: Jossey-Bass.

Horne, A. & Sayger, T. (1990). *Treating conduct and oppositional defiant disorders in children.* Pergamon Press.

Kagan, R. & Schlosberg, S. (1989). *Families in perpetual crisis.* W.W. Norton.

Kagan, S.L. & Weissbourd, B. (Eds.). (1994). *Putting families first: America's family support movement and the challenge of change.* San Francisco: Jossey-Bass.

Kahn, S. (1995). Community organization. In *The encyclopedia of social work,* 19th ed. (Vol. 1, pp. 569-576). Washington, DC: NASW Press.

Kaplan, L. & Girard, J.L. (1994). *Strengthening high-risk families: A handbook for practitioners.* New York: Lexington Books.

Kreilkamp, T. (1989). *Time-limited intermittent therapy with children and families.* New York: Brunner/Mazel.

Lacayo, R. (1996, January 15). Law and order. *Time*: 48-54.

Linton, T. E. (1971). The educateur model: A theoretical monograph. *Journal of Special Education, 5,* 2: 155-190.

Massinga, R.W. (1994). Transforming social services: Family-supportive strategies. In S.L. Kagan, & B. Weissbourd, (Eds.). *Putting families first: America's family support movement and the challenge of change.* (pp. 93-111). San Francisco: Jossey-Bass.

McCann, N. (April 22, 1998). Hattiesburg vies for All-America city. *Hattiesburg American,* Hattiesburg, Mississippi.

Mulroy, E. (1997). Building a neighborhood network: Interorganizational collaboration to prevent child abuse and neglect. *Social Work, 42,* 3: 255-264.

Mulvey, E., Arthur, M., & Reppucci, N. (1997). The prevention of juvenile delinquency: A review of the research. *The Prevention Researcher, 4,* 2: 1-4.

O'Donnell, J., Hawkins, J., Catalano, R., Abbotte, R., & Day, L. (1997). Seattle social development project: Preventing delinquency among low-income children. *The Prevention Researcher, 4,* 2: 7-9.

O'Hanlon, W.H. & Weiner-Davis, M. (1989). *In search of solutions: A new definition of psychotherapy.* New York: W.W. Norton.

Pecora, P.J., Whittaker, J.K., & Maluccio, A.N. (1992). *The child welfare challenge: Policy, practice, and research.* New York: Aldine de Gruyter.

Quinn, W., Bell, M., & Ward, B. (1997). Family solutions for juvenile first offenders. *The Prevention Researcher, 4,* 2: 10-12.

Rhodes, J.E. & Jason, L.A. (1988). *Preventing substance abuse children and adolescents.* Pergamon Press.

Schaefer, C.E., Briesmeiste, J.M., & Fitton, M.E. (1984). *Family therapy techniques for problem behaviors of children and teenagers.* San Francisco: Jossey-Bass.

Schorr, L. (1989). *Within our reach: Breaking the cycle of disadvantage.* Doubleday.

Selekman, M.D. (1996). *Pathways to change: Brief therapy solutions with difficult adolescents*. Guilford Press.

Skogan, W.G. & Wycoff, M.A. (1986). Storefront police officers: The Houston field test. In D.P. Rosenbaum (Ed.), *Community crime prevention: Does it work?* (pp. 179-199). Beverly Hills, CA: Sage.

Specht, H. & Courtney, M. (1994). *Unfaithful angels: How social work has abandoned its mission*. New York: Free Press.

Strayhorn, J. (1988). *The competent child*. New York: Guilford.

Sutphen, R. (1997). Social work and juvenile justice: Is the literature trying to tell us something? *Arete*, *22*, 1: 50-57.

Thornberry, T., Huizinga, D., & Loeber, R. (1995). The prevention of serious delinquency and violence. In J.C. Howell, B. Krisberg, J. Hawkins, & J. Wilson (Eds.), *Serious, violent, & chronic juvenile offender: A sourcebook*. (pp. 213-237). Sage Publications.

Thurman, Q.C. (1995). Community policing: The police as a community resource. In P. Adams and K. Nelson (Eds.), *Reinventing human services: Community- and family-centered practice*. New York: Aldine de Gruyter.

Treger, H. (1987). The police social work team. In W.G. Bailey (Ed.), *The encyclopedia of police science* (pp. 48-486). New York: Garland.

Treger, H. (1995). Police social work. In *The Encyclopedia of Social Work*, 19th ed. (Vol. 3, pp. 1843-1848). Washington, D.C.: NASW Press.

United States General Accounting Office. (1996, March). *At risk and delinquent youth: Multiple federal programs raise efficiency questions*. Washington, DC. U.S. General Accounting Office.

Vorrath, H. & Brendtro, L. (1985). *Positive peer culture* (2nd edition). New York: Aldine.

Whittaker., J.K. (1980). *Caring for troubled children*. San Francisco: Jossey-Bass.

Collaborative Practice in Low Income Communities: University, Agency, Public School Partnerships

Cathryne L. Schmitz

SUMMARY. Children and families in high risk low income communities are facing increasing stress due to rising poverty, increasing violence and isolation, and decreasing resources. Community based, family support centers are nationally recognized as vital in serving high risk communities. Yet, successful collaborative ventures are difficult, funding is problematic, and informed evaluation is elusive. This article will review the efforts of leaders in local government and business to come together with faculty from an urban university, public education, private non-profit family serving agencies, and child advocates to build centers through a recommitment of resources. The role of the university in the development, implementation, and evaluation of community collaboratives is presented. Cross-site comparison allows a discussion of

---

Cathryne L. Schmitz, PhD, ACSW, LCSW, is affiliated with the Graduate School of Social Work, University of Denver, 2148 South High Street, Denver, CO 80208 (E-mail: cschmitz@du.edu).

The author would like to thank the Family Resource Center and Youth in Need for their contributions to the community through quality services provided in these school-linked services. Their work made this article possible. Thanks as well to The Missouri Department of Public Safety for financial support of two sites through the Delinquency and Youth Violence Prevention Program and the U.S. Department of Health and Human Services Office of Community Services for their support of the third site through the Family Support Center and Gateway Demonstration Programs.

[Haworth co-indexing entry note]: "Collaborative Practice in Low Income Communities: University, Agency, Public School Partnerships." Schmitz, Cathryne L. Co-published simultaneously in *Social Thought* (The Haworth Pastoral Press, an imprint of The Haworth Press, Inc.) Vol. 19, No. 2, 1999, pp. 53-67; and: *Raising Our Children Out of Poverty* (ed: John J. Stretch et al.) The Haworth Pastoral Press, an imprint of The Haworth Press, Inc., 1999, pp. 53-67. Single or multiple copies of this article are available for a fee from The Haworth Document Delivery Service [1-800-342-9678, 9:00 a.m. - 5:00 p.m. (EST). E-mail address: getinfo@haworthpressinc.com].

the factors contributing to successful collaboration. *[Article copies available for a fee from The Haworth Document Delivery Service: 1-800-342-9678. E-mail address: getinfo@haworthpressinc.com <Website: http://www.haworthpressinc.com>]*

KEYWORDS. Collaboration, child poverty, interdisciplinary, high risk communities

Rising rates of poverty and violence place children in the United States (U.S.) at growing risk. With child poverty increasing by a third between 1969 (14%) and 1997 (21%), children in the U.S. experience higher rates of poverty (Children's Defense Fund [CDF], 1997) than children in any other industrialized nation. Children, now twice as likely to live in poverty as adults (11%), are the nation's poorest segment. This increased poverty has resulted in increased stress for children, families, and sometimes whole communities.

The U.S. is also "among the most violent nations in the world" (Brueggemann, 1996, p. 34) with the "highest homicide rate of any industrialized nation" (DeCuevas, 1992, p. 48). In spite of the current concern about adolescents as perpetrators of crime, our children are ten times more likely to be victims rather than perpetrators of crime (CDF, 1997) with studies indicating a heightened concern for inner-city youth. A Chicago study found that 44% of children and youth had witnessed a shooting, 33% witnessed a stabbing, and 25% witnessed a murder (Garbarino, Kostelny, & Dubrow, 1991).

While poverty presents the greatest risk to children (CDF, 1994; McWhirter, McWhirter, McWhirter, & McWhirter, 1993), stress is increased when multiple risk factors interact (Schorr, 1988). Job loss, substandard housing, an inadequate education system, and flight from the city of those with resources worsens with the economic crisis increasing the risk and trauma (Alter, Deutelbaum, Dodd, Else, & Raheim, 1992). The stress is often reflected through a negative impact on the school performance of children (CDF, 1994; Dupper & Poertner, 1997) with the multitude of obstacles presented by economically and socially disadvantaged environments contributing to "the development of a variety of emotional, behavioral, and cognitive disorders" (Catron & Weiss, 1994, p. 247). Intervention targeted at reducing some of the risk factors can reduce the negative outcomes (Schorr). At a time when neighborhoods with the highest level of distress need the best resources, they are likely to have the fewest resources (Nelson, 1995).

School programs providing a supportive climate and positive regard have demonstrated the potential for a significant impact on high risk children (McWhirter et al., 1993; Schorr, 1988). The development of programs providing supportive, stimulating environments helps children compensate for early risk (Schorr, 1988) but the issues are complex for children experiencing learning and performance difficulties at school. Schools cannot function successfully unless the social and emotional factors impacting youth are addressed (Adelman & Taylor, 1993, p. 32). "Traditional programs face limitations" (Resnick, Burt, Newmark, & Reilly, 1992, p. vii) in meeting these needs. Community-based human service efforts, however, have been identified as a promising service model for communities affected by poverty (Mulroy, 1997).

School-linked services are vital in communities struggling with child poverty and related social issues (Hare, 1995); and programs designed to link a range of social and health services to the schools are increasingly recognized as promising (Dupper & Poertner, 1997). They provide the opportunity for pooling resources and addressing inter-related social, economic, education, and health factors (Pires-Hester, 1990). While the schools provide a logical location for meeting the complex needs of high risk children and families, they do not have the resources to assist families with the complexity of their needs; collaborative development and service delivery is required (Caplan & Gal, 1996). This has resulted in increased attention focused on integrated, collaborative, comprehensive service models (Mason, 1997; Resnick et al., 1992). They provide the opportunity for pooling resources and addressing inter-related social, economic, education, and health factors (Pires-Hester, 1990). Although a comprehensive approach is needed to meet the needs of high risk youth, collaborations are difficult, pulling against the perceived self-need of agencies (Dryfoos, 1990).

The discussion of the need to form linkages as a basis for school reform is not new (Franklin & Streeter, 1995). Progressive educators called for the development of comprehensive schools which included a range of human services to address school reform needs at the turn of the century and again in the 1960s. Unfortunately, the bureaucratic management model grew out of the call for change early in the century. The 1960s call for decentralization and inclusion led to the alternative school movement (Franklin & Streeter). Over time, a tension has developed between the pull for centralized control within the school system and the push to reach outward. This tension provides the backdrop for the current attempts at linking services across systems (Franklin & Streeter).

Approaches to linkage and collaboration vary widely. Litwak and Rothman (1970) defined three models of interorganizational practice (formal, coordination, linkage) based on the strength of the formality. Formal structures call for rules, linkages rely on coordinating mechanisms rather than rules, and informal groups rely on contacts between agencies involved. Moving beyond coordination which "implies a concerted effort to work together," collaboration "implies the concept of a joint venture" (Netting, Kettner, & McMurtry, 1993, p. 112). A loose collaboration, formed when organizations with primary allegiances outside the collaboration work together informally to meet a common goal, is generally referred to a coalition. Sometimes a coalition, formed on a temporary basis to meet immediate needs, will discover the benefits of ongoing collaboration (Brody & Nair, 1997; Netting et al.).

One conceptual model for defining collaboration is provided by Germain (1984) and reviewed by Bope and Jost (1994). The common forms according to this model are conferring, cooperating, consulting, multiple entry, and team work. Franklin and Streeter (1995) define five models: informal relations, coordination, partnerships, collaboration, and integration. These models provide a continuum of commitment from little to significant.

Drawing on the five components presented by Germain (1984) and the combined features of collaboration and integration as defined by Franklin and Streeter (1995), the model used for the development of the collaboratives reviewed in this article builds from shared leadership, comprehensive planning, redistribution of resources, and interdisciplinary teamwork. In line with Mokuau and Ewalt (1993) three key factors undergirded the collaborative vision: (a) shared governance, (b) interdisciplinary care, and (c) multicultural perspective. The comprehensive model developed and evaluated followed the family resource center collaborative model with school-linked integration of a broad range of services including health, recreation, mental health, employment, education, and basic needs (Dupper & Poertner, 1997).

Collaboration among families and community institutions including schools has been shown to provide high risk children with a sense of belonging and hope (McWhirter et al., 1993; Schorr, 1988). These "efforts can mobilize the energy and resources within each of the separate sectors, and provide the high quality, comprehensive services children and families need to go as far as their talents and industry will take them" (Melaville & Blank, 1991, p. 36). Those attempting to develop collaborative school-linked services, however, are faced with multiple challenges including funding, space, turf, resistance, and structures such as confidentiality (Dupper & Poertner, 1997). Agencies tend to operate independently maintaining control over decision making and resources (Brody & Nair, 1997). Contractual agreements help prevent disintegration of structures designed to provide and maintain comprehensive access whether through task forces, committees, or coalitions (Dryfoos, 1990).

Practice wisdom indicates that a number of factors contribute to the successful development of collaborative ventures. Included are (a) mutual trust and a shared vision (Mulroy, 1997); (b) careful selection of partners providing complementary resources and skills (Groark & McCall, 1996; Matheny, 1994); (c) healthy communication patterns, time management, and interpersonal skills (Osterloh & Koorland, 1998); and (d) committed leadership (U.S. Dept. of Education, 1995). Although family support centers are entrenched in the literature as effective, there is little research on either the development process of community-based services (Mulroy) or the specific leadership qualities required to facilitate successful collaboration. This review of the development and implementation of three centers begins a process of analyzing the development process through comparative analysis across three sites.

DEVELOPMENT

As Goetz and Peck (1994) outline, family support services offer hope for the development of more effective centers for vulnerable children. The wisdom from the review of effective centers indicates the necessity for (a) collaborative, cross-systems development, (b) interagency involvement, (c) participation of all players from the beginning of the development process, (d) shared goals and vision, and (e) realistic evaluation.

In this mid-sized, midwestern city, business leaders, private nonprofit organizations, governmental agencies, public school staff, university representatives, and community members including parents and youth came together to discuss their concerns about the growing risk facing children and families. With a child poverty rate of 39.9%–up from 33.7% in 1980 (Citizens for Missouri's Children [CMC], 1995) and increasing racial isolation with many resources continuing to move from the city to the surrounding areas, the public schools and the children and families served were struggling.

Two parallel processes came together (see Table 1). The public schools moved to integrate 15 of their schools (elementary and middle schools) into the local communities through the development of community education centers (CEC). At the same time, provider agencies came together with other invested community resources to develop family centered, community based, collaborative hubs for service delivery. The collaborative nature was reflected in the grant writing process which involved members of the community in an effort to design programs that met locally identified needs. The goal was to produce family support centers based on the needs expressed by the neighborhood.

The Neighborhoods

Three neighborhoods[1] with multiple risk factors for families with children were chosen for network development. These neighborhoods exhibited high poverty and unemployment rates as well as high rates of crime, school dropout, and levels of unemployment among youth (see Table 2). The population in two of these neighborhoods is dropping and few housing units are owner occupied. Two of the neighborhoods were chosen because of extreme racial isolation (Roosevelt and Cornell); the other (Washington) was more ethnically/racially diverse. The youth in all three schools are at very high risk with 98% of the students qualifying for the free lunch program.

TABLE 1. The Merging of Dual Tracks

Public Education	Child Advocacy Networks
Players: Public Schools Community Education Centers Local Community *Goal:* Integrate the public schools into their surrounding communities *Process:* Develop councils from the surrounding community comprised of parents, youth, neighborhood, residents, local organizations, local political leaders Assess community need and desires Enlist commitment from residents and organizations for resources and services Develop responsive programs	*Players*: Business/Industry Private Nonprofits University Public Systems Child Advocates *Goal:* Develop neighborhood based, family centered and family inclusive, strength based, interdisciplinary hubs for service delivery with a recommitment of local funds and minimal grant support *Process:* Ongoing collaborative process to identify resources for interdisciplinary programs Enlist commitment from local providers and service systems Identify sites with high risk factors

TABLE 2. Neighborhood Risk Factors*

	Roosevelt	Washington	Cornell	National
Child Poverty	67.4%	50.1%	59%	21.2%
Free/Reduced Lunch	98%	98%	98%	24%
Teen Birthrate	29.8%	17.9%	33%	8.6%
Kids at Risk of Hunger	89.7%	64%	64%	25%
Low Birthweight Babies	21.17%	11.38%	18%	7%
Late/No Prenatal Care	24%	11.7%	44%	6.1%
Child Abuse/Neg/1000	114.3	86.1	97.5	25.5
Vacant House Units	27.5%	22.5%	12%	15.4% (city)
16-19y-no sch/diploma	27.67%	44%	32%	17.5%
Unemployment	23.7%	14.3%	15.5%	6.8%
Current Population	93% black 7% white	43% black 55% white 2% Asian	92% black 8% white	12% black** 73% white 4% Asian 10%Hispanic 1% Am. Indian

(*Data from Project Respond, 1993,1995 unless noted; **U.S. Dept. of Commerce, 1997)

Roosevelt had one of the highest rates of reported drug sales in the city. The neighborhood also exhibited high rates of homicide, robbery, and aggravated assault as well as moderate rates of burglary, larceny, and auto theft. Washington experienced one of the highest rates of larceny, burglary, and destruction of property as well as high rates of robbery, aggravated assault, auto theft, and reported drug sales along with moderate rates of homicide. Cornell was also a high crime area with gang activity in the area surrounding the school, and a high incidence of child and youth crime victims. (Data provided by the public school system.)

Vision

Two networks were responsible for the development of the three sites. The centers at Roosevelt and Washington (based in elementary schools) were developed by an ongoing, child advocacy network. The center at Cornell (based in a middle school) was developed by a network brought together to develop this collaborative school-linked service. The networks envisioned family and child centered services embedded within the CEC (see Figure 1). The CECs, designed to help integrate the public schools into their surrounding communities, provide an ideal setting for collaborative programming.

A two-pronged strategy was employed to improve family functioning, school achievement, community development, and school family connections. The family support centers involved a plan for coordinated service delivery with linkage to community resources. At each site, a mixture of enrichment and counseling/case management services was provided. Services were designed to be (a) family focused/family friendly services, (b) strength based, (c) culturally appropriate, and (d) community driven. These centers were funded through state and federal grants with a shifting commitment of resources by local agencies.

IMPLEMENTATION

The family support centers at Roosevelt and Washington began in January 1995; the third one followed the next year. The programs focused on increasing effective management within families, family commitment to school, academic success, and high school completion rate as well as decreasing family conflict. In order to meet these goals, the sites developed systems for parent outreach, counseling/case management, child development training, conflict resolution and violence prevention, and linking families with other CEC and community services. In addition, tutoring and other resources were expanded.

FIGURE 1. Model of Collaborative Imbedding

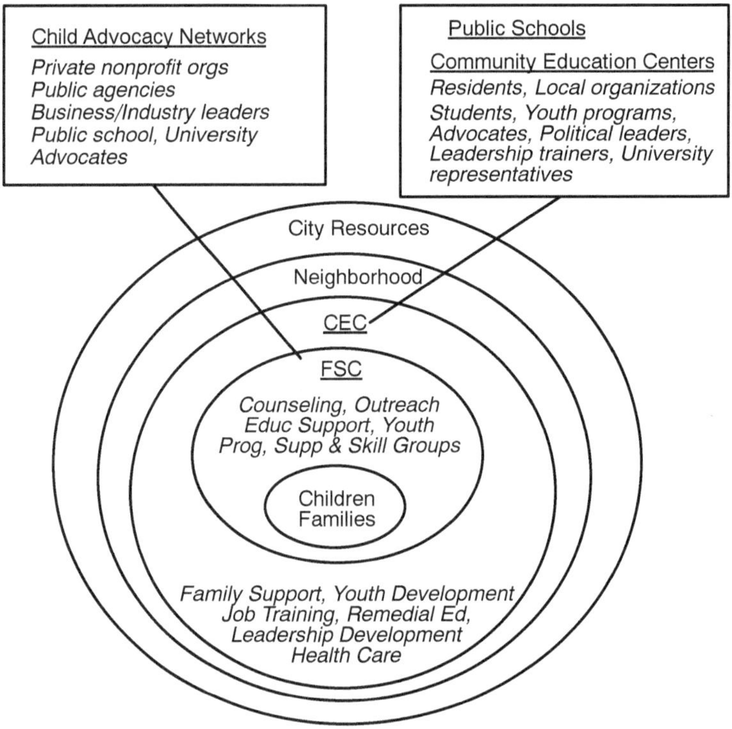

The specific components developed at each center were multi-disciplinary, multi-system, and multi-agency and based on an assessment of neighborhood residents and school personnel. The following components were identified as primary program needs: (a) health/mental health; (b) learning support; (c) economic well-being/job skills; (d) self-improvement; (e) afternoon, evening, and week-end programming; and (f) basic service (housing, child care, etc.) linkage. The initial components of the centers included parent outreach, home based family counseling, outreach case management, parent training, training of school personnel, youth tutoring, and skill development for children, youth, and adults. Substance abuse prevention, adult education/employment, and primary health care were incorporated as needed/available.

Coordinating collaborative implementation, administration/supervision, and service delivery was complex. Regular administrative meetings involving school, agency, and university personnel were instituted to deal with administrative, service, and staff related implementation issues. Participatory evaluation, incorporated from the beginning, provided feedback to the administrative team allowing for changes in the implementation process. Hiring was coordinated with the inclusion of agency and school personnel.

EVALUATION

The evaluation of complex, interdisciplinary collaboratives requires the use of dynamic, multi-method inquiry (Mulroy & Shay, 1997). Participatory action research (as described by Patton, 1990) facilitated the duality of evaluation and implementation. Evaluation of the centers was provided by an interdisciplinary (social work and education) team from a city based university. The evaluation was designed collaboratively with the centers and community and involved action research with process and outcome components. Process evaluation measured the collaborative process, program development, and service integration. Interviews and focus groups with youth, families, and school personnel along with participant observation were used to gather data. Outcome data was gathered through referral forms, intake assessment, and agency and academic records as well as interviews of youth, families, and staff at the schools and family support centers. Service delivery, impact of services, and attitudes of youth, families, and school personnel were measured. Evaluators also participated in administrative, development, and implementation meetings; observed services; and interviewed participants. The findings helped shape the implementation of the centers.

Results

Baseline data gathered through focus groups and interviews provided information on attitudes and concerns. The collaborative team members (supervisors from the schools and agencies) had a vision for the school, children, and community. They were hopeful but also had concerns about resources, turf, and time. Early difficulties surrounded communication, coordination, and funding.

The teachers, youth, and families were unaware of the developing programs. Overall, the teachers were negative about the school, children, and families. The youth had ideas for programming and marketing. They wanted safety, role models, and respectful communication. They expressed concern about teen parents and were worried that "people don't seem to care." The adult community members interviewed were concerned about teen mothers as well as the lack of resources. They saw a need for skill training and afterschool programs.

Interviews at the end of years two and three indicated changes in attitude and knowledge. The teachers were more positive about the school, children, and families. The youth, families, and teachers knew about the range of programs at the school including the family support centers. The collaborative team felt positive about the relationships and services/resources developed, but the time commitment required for collaborative services was still of concern. At each site, the role of leadership, communication patterns, and turf issues was discussed. Funding accessibility continued to be problematic at Roosevelt and Washington where the money was funneled through the school district. It was not a concern at Cornell where the funds moved through the private, non-profit agency.

A range of services and resources were provided across the sites (see Table 3). Supplies such as copying and fax equipment, and at one site, a van, enriched the programs and facilitated community outreach. Tutoring support contributed across the sites. Counseling, outreach, and case management services were provided. Enrichment programs included camping, youth job training, computer classes, recreation, arts programs, video evening, Kwanzaa celebrations, dances, Double Dutch with leadership training, adult education, and a family chili dinner. The van was effective in increasing accessibility. Regular, dependable transportation increased security. Outreach case management was much more effective at engaging families than school based family counseling. Parent outreach, which involved the early recruitment of parents in building the program and engaging other parents, was very effective at increasing parent participation. At Cornell, where there had not been a parent association for 10 years, the use of parents to build programs established a growing parent program. The chili dinner was attended by 75 families.

Findings and Implications

The centers based development on the principles outlined in the literature. A common purpose, shared mission and purpose, and agreement on projects (Groark & McCall, 1996) provided a foundation. There were varying levels of success, however. Leadership style, communication patterns, personalities and attitudes, and funding determined the ease or difficulty experienced by the partners as they moved from development into implementation.

Basic personalities were a key factor. The embedding of the projects within a dynamic system meant success was partially based on the ability of the staff and administrators to tolerate controlled chaos. Most disruptive were individuals unable to share power, space, and control. They were able to undermine both morale and working relationships without skillful, directed supervision.

The leader set the tone for tolerance and process. Leadership which facilitated staff in carrying out their jobs creatively and independently was central to successful development. Staff who were respected and empowered by the

TABLE 3. Descriptive Overview of Major Service Components*

SERVICES/RESOURCES & PROGRAM COMPONENTS	DESCRIPTION
Counseling/case management	School based counseling for children and youth–planned and informal; home based counseling for parents and family; case management to support families in meeting basic needs
Parent/family outreach	Para professional outreach to engage families in school and youth activities
Tutoring	After school tutoring supervised by paid trained staff with volunteer tutors
Social support	Classroom outreach, youth activities and recreation, summer camp, classes
Training	Social and activity skill training incorporated into the recreational, educational, social activities
Recreation	Social support and skill training including conflict resolution provided through organized and informal recreational activities.
Youth activities	Dances; earn-a-bike (youth earn their bike through a bike education and program teaching responsibility and social skills); trips to the mall earned through participation and designed to teach social skills; double Dutch team providing an opportunity for skill building, success, and esteem building provided with a requirement for participation in tutoring and leadership development (won championship); ongoing computer courses teaching computer and educational skills; sewing classes
Youth Corp	Work and social skill training; conflict resolution
Youth mentors	Older youth mentor younger youth
Summer enrichment	Kindergarten success (for youth who needed additional instruction to pass kindergarten); Art Program (intensive workshop run by an artist and a human service staff; taught education and social skill; provided a successful activity designing and completing a wall mural)
Camp programs	Summer day camps providing education, recreation, social development, and field activities exposing the youth to a range of experiences; overnight camps for youth and families designed to expand experiences, teach skills, and work on family relationships
Teen parent program	Intensive ongoing support and skill training offered from pregnancy and into parenting
Family activities	Designed to provide positive parent and family interaction with the school and increase parent participation and involvement; activities included the formation of a core parent group which developed events including Kwanzaa celebrations, a chili dinner with 250 families, a family skating party, and the development of a PTA for the first time in 10 years
Adult education & employment training	Designed to help parents and young adults in meeting their goals
Resources	To support program development and operation included office equipment (fax, copiers, computers) and at 1 site a van which facilitated programming, family involvement, and youth safety in returning home
Staff training	Support for staff to increase knowledge and skills
Graduate interns	Program support and skill development; participated in service delivery and evaluation

*Categories are overlapping

leader to operate with flexibility developed trust and a "can do" attitude. Successful leadership also involved the ability to take control and negotiate staff process when difficult issues arose. With strong leadership, teams were able to overcome the communication and turf difficulties at one site.

Some variables were beyond the control of the collaborative. Partnership selection was recognized as important (Groark & McCall, 1996) and initial decisions were carefully processed. Given the dynamic nature of the sites, however, partners changed. The change in principals at Cornell provided a leadership which was highly successful. On the other hand, there were partners added to the CECs which disrupted the collaboratives.

Open, respectful communication tolerant of conflict, with clear channels established by the leader laid the foundation for functional collegial relationships. The significance of a liaison person in facilitating cross-site communication (Groark & McCall, 1996) was confirmed. The lack of a liaison at Roosevelt and Washington was a major gap, undermining many efforts. Finally, this study confirmed the role of attitudes and resources in the success or failure of collaborative ventures (Groark & McCall, 1996). The vision of the collaborative partners facilitated the development which led to changes in attitudes in school personnel.

Resources positively impacted programming with the van leading to increased success with youth and families. In addition, accessibility of funding had a major impact. Placement within a large bureaucracy increased turf battles and restricted access. Funds funneled through the large school district were much less accessible than funds funneled through the mid-sized private, non-profit family serving agency. Accessibility of funds for the development of enrichment programs designed based on site need allowed the development of a range of programs increasing program use by children and youth as well as interaction with the families.

CONCLUSION

Collaborative, creative commitment is required if we are to provide children and youth from impoverished communities with the same educational opportunities available to more advantaged children and youth (Annie E. Casey, 1997). No one model of school-linked services exists. This makes it necessary for localities to build programs tailored for their needs, based on the lessons learned from existing programs (Levy & Shepardson, 1992). In that vein, the collaborative, school-based services highlighted were designed by communities attempting to address the needs of their highest risk youth and families. Services were individualized and tailored to meet the specific needs of the neighborhood. Success was largely dependent on leadership style, attitudes, communication patterns, personalities, and access to funding. Funding flexibility and accessibility was imperative.

Interdisciplinary and university-community relationships can expand the resources. The university has the potential to contribute site and technological resources; faculty expertise with the provision consultation and evaluation; and student commitment through their involvement in service delivery as well as the evaluative process. Some universities, particularly those strategically placed within or near high risk communities, have begun to examine their roles and responsibility to come together for the benefit of the children.

Education and social work provide complementary knowledge and expertise. The social work profession, with its history of involvement in community development within impoverished communities, has the knowledge and experience needed to facilitate the creative development of school-linked services (Dupper & Poertner, 1997; Franklin & Streeter, 1995). The combining of university, education, and human service resources, knowledge, and expertise can result in the development of services effective in (a) helping children and youth experiencing difficulties, (b) increasing family involvement, and (c) developing neighborhood centers for enrichment and development. These kinds of services have the potential to help meet the needs of the nation's children. The lessons learned here provide a basis for understanding the beginning stages of development and implementation. Without an ongoing commitment of funding, however, programs cannot maintain their commitment.

NOTE

1. The names used for the neighborhoods/schools are fictitious and have no relationship to existing schools by those names.

REFERENCES

Adelman, H. S. & Taylor, L. (1993). School-based mental health: Toward a comprehensive approach. *Journal of Mental Health Administration*, *20*, 32-45.

Alter, C., Deutelbaum, W., Dodd, T. E., Else, J., & Raheim, S. (1992, March). *Integrating three strategies of family empowerment: Family, community, and economic development*. Paper presented at the annual program meeting of the Council on Social Work Education, Kansas City, MO.

Annie E. Casey Foundation. (1997). *Kids count data book: State profiles of child well-being*. Baltimore, MD: Author.

Bope, E. T. & Jost, T. S. (1994). Interprofessional collaboration: Factors that affect form, function, and structure. In R. M. Casto, M. C. Julia, L. J. Platt, G. L. Harbaugh, W. R. Waugaman, A. Thompson, T. S. Jost, E. T. Bope, T. Williams, & D. B. Lee, *Interprofessional care and collaborative practice* (pp. 61-69). Pacific Grove, CA: Brooks/Cole Publishing Company.

Brody, R. & Nair, M. D. (1997). *Macro practice: A generalist approach.* Wheaton, IL: Gregory Publishing Company.

Brueggemann, W. G. (1996). *The practice of macro social work.* Chicago, IL: Nelson-Hall Publishers.

Caplan, J. & Gal, A. (1996). The school: The crossroads for collaboration. *Journal of Children and Poverty, 2*, 55-64.

Catron, T. & Weiss, B. (1994). The Vanderbilt School-based Counseling Program: An interagency, primary-care model of mental health services. *Journal of Emotional and Behavioral Disorders, 2*, 247-253).

Children's Defense Fund. (1994). *Wasting America's future.* Boston, MA: Beacon Press.

Children's Defense Fund. (1997). *The state of America's children: Yearbook 1997.* Washington, DC: Author.

Citizens for Missouri's Children. (1995). *Kids Count Missouri: 1995 Report.* St. Louis, MO: Author.

DeCuevas, J. (1992). Our children are in trouble. *Harvard Magazine, 95* (1), 46-53.

Dryfoos, J. G. (1990). *Adolescents at risk: Prevalence and prevention.* New York: Oxford University Press.

Dupper, D. R. & Poertner. (1997). Public schools and the revitalization of impoverished communities: School-linked, family resource centers. *Social Work, 42*, 415-422.

Franklin, C. & Streeter, C. L. (1995). School reform: Linking public schools with human services. *Social Work, 40*, 773-782.

Garbarino, J., Kostelny, K. & Dubrow, N. (1991). *No place to be a child: Growing up in a war zone.* Lexington, MA: Lexington Books.

Germain, C. B. (1984). *Social work practice in health care: An ecological perspective.* New York: The Free Press.

Goetz, K. & Peck, S. (Eds.). (1994). *The basics of family support: A guide for state planners (and others).* Chicago, IL: Family Resource Coalition.

Groark, C. J. & McCall, R. B. (1996). Building successful university-community human service agency collaborations. In C. B. Fisher, J. P. Murray, & I. E. Sigel (Eds.). *Applied developmental science: Graduate training for diverse disciplines and educational settings* (pp. 237-251). Norwood, NJ: Ablex.

Hare, I. (1995) School-linked services. In *Encyclopedia of Social Work* (19th ed., pp. 2100-2109). Washington, DC: NASW Press.

Levy, J. E. & Shepardson, W. (1992). A school at current school-linked service efforts. In R. E. Behrman (Ed.), *The future of children, 2* (1). Los Altos, CA: Center for the Future of Children.

Litwak, E. & Rothman, J. (1970). Towards the theory and practice of coordination between formal organizations. in W. P. Rosengren & M. Lipton, *Organizations and clients: Essays in the sociology of service* (pp. 137-186). Columbus, OH: Charles E. Merrill Publishing Company.

McWhirter, J. J., McWhirter, B. T., McWhirter, A. M., & McWhirter, E. H. (1993). *At risk youth: A comprehensive response.* Pacific Grove, CA: Brooks/Cole.

Mason, V. L. (1997). Leaping across the American paradox: Why I believe we can change the way America works for families. *Family Support Council Newsletter, 2* (2), 2.

Matheny, P. (1994). Collaborative partnerships involving the community. *Journal of Health Administration Education, 12* (3), 281-290.

Melaville, A. I. & Blank, M. J. (1991). *What it takes: Structuring interagency partnerships to connect children and families with comprehensive services.* Washington, DC: Education and Human Services Consortium.

Mokuau, N. & Ewalt, P. L. (1993). School-agency collaboration: Enriching teaching, scholarship, and service in state hospital placements. *Journal of Social Work Education, 29*, 328-337.

Mulroy, E. A. (1997). Building a neighborhood network: Interorganizational collaboration to prevent child abuse and neglect. *Social Work, 42*, 255-264.

Mulroy, E. A. & Shay, S. (1997). Nonprofit organizations and innovation: A model of neighborhood-based collaboration to prevent child maltreatment. *Social Work, 42*, 515-524.

Nelson, D. W. (1995). Investing in the future: Rescue plans for children at risk. *The National Voter, 44* (2), 14-15, 18.

Netting, F. E., Kettner, P. M., & McMurtry, S. L. (1993). *Social work macro practice.* New York: Longman.

Osterloh, A. E. & Koorland, M. A. (1997). Working together: Mental health and special education collaboration in Florida. In C. J. Liberton, K. Kutash, & R. M. Friedman (Eds.), *10th annual research conference proceedings: A system of care for children's mental health: Expanding the research base*, (pp. 151-154).

Patton, M. Q. (1992). *Qualitative evaluation and research methods* (2nd ed.). Newbury Park, CA: Sage Publications.

Pires-Hester, L. J. (1990, December). *School-based health clinics in an "education" society.* Paper presented at the meeting of the Third Annual Conference on Universities, Community Schools and Job Training, Philadelphia, PA.

Project Respond (1993). *The children of metropolitan St. Louis 1993: A report to the community.* St. Louis, MO: Author.

Project Respond (1995). *The children of metropolitan St. Louis 1995: A report to the community.* St. Louis, MO: Author.

Resnick, G., Burt, M. R., Newmark, L., & Reilly, L. (1995) *Youth at risk: Definitions, prevalence, and approaches to service delivery.* (Contract No: HHS-100-92-0005). Washington, DC: Urban Institute.

Schorr, L. B. (1988). *Within our reach: Breaking the cycle of disadvantage.* New York: Doubleday.

U.S. Department of Commerce. (1997). *Statistical abstract of the United States 1997* (117th edition). Washington, DC: U.S. Government Printing Office.

U.S. Department of Education, Office of Educational Research and Improvement, Educational Resources Information Center. (1995). *School-linked comprehensive services for children and families: What we know and what we need to know.* (Report No. Ed 1.302:SCH 6/22). Washington, DC: Office of Educational Research and Improvement. (ERIC Document Reproduction Service No. ED 382580).

Weiss, H. & Halpern, R. (1991). *Community-based family support and education programs: Something old or something new*? NY: National Center for Children in Poverty.

Fostering Resiliency in Children: Lessons Learned in Transcending Adversity

Nancie Palmer

SUMMARY. The centerpiece of this presentation is the Differential Resiliency Model [DRM], an original conceptual framework developed by the author to promote understanding of the process of "survival" and the development of resilience over time. Drawing on the DRM, practitioners and other helping advocates may more adequately and timely identify and intervene with appropriate resources. Approaching children in poverty and adversity with a new appreciation for their capacity and strengths may also enhance their growth to a level of thriving. It is not enough to settle for "survival" or a "good enough" quality of life. The ultimate test is enabling children and their families to thrive and flourish. It is the *only* acceptable standard of professional and social response. *[Article copies available for a fee from The Haworth Document Delivery Service: 1-800-342-9678. E-mail address: getinfo@haworthpressinc.com <Website: http://www.haworthpressinc.com>]*

KEYWORDS. Social advocacy, social resilience, strengths perspective, social development, ecological perspective

PROLOGUE

Smoke curls forlornly upward from the silhouette gazing out the window. Chance would be coming home soon. Chance, one of six brothers, third youngest. The silhouette sighs and pours herself another drink. Her aching despair envelops the room. It's been this way, forever.

Nancie Palmer, PhD, ACSW, is Chair, Department of Social Work, Washburn University.

[Haworth co-indexing entry note]: "Fostering Resiliency in Children: Lessons Learned in Transcending Adversity." Palmer, Nancie. Co-published simultaneously in *Social Thought* (The Haworth Pastoral Press, an imprint of The Haworth Press, Inc.) Vol. 19, No. 2, 1999, pp. 69-87; and: *Raising Our Children Out of Poverty* (ed: John J. Stretch et al.) The Haworth Pastoral Press, an imprint of The Haworth Press, Inc., 1999, pp. 69-87. Single or multiple copies of this article are available for a fee from The Haworth Document Delivery Service [1-800-342-9678, 9:00 a.m. - 5:00 p.m. (EST). E-mail address: getinfo@haworthpressinc.com].

Down the road, Chance sees his mother. "A beacon in the window," he muses in an interview with this researcher. When she died prematurely from cirrhosis of the liver, he was "devastated." The impact from this loss has been constant though grief and loss are all too familiar to him. He reports having lost seven peers to accidents and suicide. Alcohol and drugs are the common threads that bonded them all. Now the silhouette has been replaced by her son who measures time in a blue haze of "hash" and "booze." Another casualty to poverty and alcohol. Another child at risk. Another statistic affirming the seemingly unbeatable odds of surviving in a poor and challenging environment.

"A growing number of clinicians and researchers are now arguing that the risk-factor model burdens at-risk children with the expectation that they will fail, and ignores those who beat the odds" (Butler, 1997, p. 25). This paper introduces the Differential Resiliency Model (DRM) that was developed and researched by the author during her exploration of resiliency in adult children of alcoholics. This population was selected because current research and practice in the areas of substance abuse are largely grounded in pathology. The DRM is viewed as an alternative, a non-pathological approach to the study children and families who are coping daily with adversity. Drawing upon the DRM, practitioners can now in a more timely manner identify and develop resources which may help raise our children out of poverty and contribute significantly to their personal growth. We must not settle for "survival" or a "good enough" quality of life. The ultimate goal is to enable children and families to thrive and flourish. It is the *only* acceptable standard of professional and social response.

LESSON ONE: THE MODEL OF PATHOLOGY REVISITED

"In making a shift from a disease-oriented to a health-oriented model of practice, recognition must be given to some of the fundamental ways in which the disease model has shaped the view of how human beings grow and change" (Weick, 1983, p. 467). Though written over a decade ago, Weick's observation is relevant today. El-Guebaly and Offord (1977) noted that the "huge body of literature on offspring of alcoholics" focuses "primarily on the casualties" (p. 364). Felsman and Vaillant (1987), in a 40 year longitudinal study of adults, noted that "clinical language rarely includes the process of healthy adaptation" (p. 302). This assertion is echoed by others in the research of risk and invulnerability (Anthony, 1987; Antonovsky, 1985; Cowen & Work, 1988). "In an attempt to understand, anticipate, and treat the pathological, the survivors and thrivers appear to pass almost unnoticed amidst the holocaust of disadvantage and tragedies of those who succumb to it" (Anthony & Cohler, 1987, p. ix).

LESSON TWO: EARLY FINDINGS IN RISK RESEARCH

The current interest in *resiliency* appears to represent a natural evolution from earlier studies of children and adults at risk. However, risk, invulnerability, and resiliency as conceptual centerpieces are still in their initial stage of development. Murphy and Moriarty (1976) profiled at risk children who were "good copers" and identified several interpersonal factors such as cognitive flexibility and capacity, ability to express a range of emotions, and an ability to function in social relationships, as helpful to children living in at risk or adverse environments. Felsman and Vaillant (1987) determined that invulnerable children were "not super kids" but rather courageous individuals who were able to sustain and persist with life over time. Anthony (1987) discovered that the imaginative ways that children employed when coping with frightening realities were also an enhancing factor. Flach's (1988) book *Resiliency: Discovering a new strength at times of stress*, helped pave the way for other publications in the 1990s devoted to the study of "protective" and "enhancing" factors that further examined the phenomenon of resiliency.

LESSON THREE: THE DIFFERENTIAL RESILIENCY MODEL EXAMINED

The entrenchment of practice in the framework of pathology, and the corresponding lack of a language to capture such factors about resiliency, compelled this author to create a new model for understanding the life experiences of survivors of adversity. In creating the DRM, the term *differential* was selected in order to convey the idea of varying qualities and attributes that could be generally distinguished from one another. The intention was to present the concept of a *range* of related features and characteristics that were measurable in increments or degrees. The concept of *degrees* is valued because of the inherent interrelationship with living things or systems and its application to an ecological framework. It has a goodness-of-fit with the social work concept of *person-in-environment*. Furthermore, when understood in the larger context, a child's (or adult's) behaviors, thoughts, feelings, and affective state may be normalized rather than viewed as pathological.

Defining *resiliency* itself is challenging. Perhaps Butler (1997) articulated the challenge best, concluding, "like pornography, resilience is harder to define than to recognize" (p. 25). For purposes of research the author operationally defined resilience as:

> a process in which the development of substantative character is made up of greater or lesser periods of disruption and the development and use of greater or lesser competencies in life management. Essential threads that enable a person to weave cumulative life experiences into an enduring fabric of self include: behavioral and cognitive competencies, and problem-solving skills that contribute to self-enhancement, and the will to have a life better than in the past. (Palmer, 1991, p. 63)

The DRM views life on a continuum which is always *in process*. This holistic concept allows for inclusion and integration, rather than a mechanistic view of human behavior in a social context. A symmetry of perspective is offered that includes function and dysfunction, growth and deterioration, decline and regeneration. It resonates with life unfolding.

Assuming that resiliency is a process, the challenge lies in understanding people-in-motion. The model presents four categories which define the salient features of the process. The author viewed these categories as snapshots, movie stills which stop the action long enough to capture the essence of the moment. The four types or degrees of resilience are: anomic survival, regenerative resilience, adaptive resilience, and flourishing resilience. They describe the degree to which particular competencies are developed and used consistently by the individual (Figure 1) and draw heavily from the natural sciences reflecting the vast restorative forces in nature (Saleebey, 1996).

Anomic survival reflects the life patterns of individuals or families who *live-on-the-edge* of destruction. Life is always in a constant state of disruption with no respite from crisis. Consistent use of dysfunctional coping behaviors is observed. Energy is directed to survival and safety.

Regenerative resilience reflects the formative development of competence and constructive coping strategies or the learning of new, more effective ways of addressing life challenges. Although the integration and internalization of these new skills and responses is tenuous, progress is sufficient enough to provide a measure of respite from crisis and an initial ability to begin to access helpful or supportive resources from the environment.

Adaptive resilience refers to relatively sustained periods of regular and extended use of competencies and constructive coping strategies such that one is able to elicit a greater degree of reciprocity between self and environment. This sustained condition provides not only essential resources for growth and change but is believed to free up one's psychic or spiritual energy for continual personal enhancement.

Flourishing resilience is illustrative of Maslow's "self-actualized" individuals (Zastrow & Kirst-Ashmen, 1990). With extended periods of stability and balance, growth and an enduring reciprocal relationship with the environment are maintained. Energy is maximized and a prevailing sense of coherence is evident.

Four life domains were used to capture significant areas of life functioning: (1) *homeostasis,* (2) *coping strategies,* (3) *relationship to environment,* and (4) *use of energy.* These domains are consistent with the social work concepts of person-in-environment, concern with social functioning, the relationship and impact of environment, and the notion of reciprocity as requisite for all living things to sustain themselves, live, repair and grow. The last domain, energy, was specifically developed because it is rarely included in the professional literature. As a life force, energy is absolutely essential.

FIGURE 1. Differential Resiliency Model

Major Life Areas				
Type of Resilience[1]	Homeostasis (Disruption and Balance)	Coping Strategies (Development and Internalization)	Relationship to Environment (Distancing and Accessing)	Use of Energy
Anomic survival	Constant state of crisis and disruption Continued need for repair	Little or no use of constructive coping strategies Consistent use of dysfunctional coping behaviors	Destructive cognitions and behaviors Diminished access to personal and environmental resources	Energy directed to survival and safety Little or no coherence or predictability to life
Regenerative resilience	Periods of some stability Crisis and disruption frequent Limited repair achieved	Formative development of constructive coping strategies Little integration and internalization	Sporadic constructive cognitions and behaviors Initiation of access to personal and environmental resources	Exceeding survival and safety needs frees energy for learning and integration Insight into self
Adaptive resilience	Sustained periods of stability and balance Some disruption, reassembly for growth	Regular use of competencies and coping strategies Some skills building needed Some integration and internalization	Regular use of competencies results in reciprocity between personal and environmental resources for growth and change	Reciprocity provides continual flow of energy to sustain birth of philosophical self
Flourishing resilience	Extended periods of stability and balance Sustained growth	Sustained use of effective cognitive and behavioral coping strategies Skills integrated and internalized	Enduring reciprocity and confidence between self and environment Flow of energy	Sense of coherence in life, enduring philosophical self Energy maximized

[1]Resilience is an evolving process. Movement is incremental but not linear. While displaying predominant characteristics of one type of resilience, a person may develop through growth of new challenges, characteristics associated with another type of resilience.
Source: Palmer, N. (1991). *Exploring resiliency in adult children of alcoholics*. p. 116. Doctoral dissertation, University of Kansas, Lawrence.

"Energy is the ability to do work. It is the force that moves things, including atoms, molecules, cellular processes, consciousness, and bodies of all shapes sizes, from planets to toes" (Pearsall, P., 1998, p. 40).

LESSON FOUR: FINDINGS HIGHLIGHTED

The challenge of capturing the "what" and "how" of surviving through adversity is a formidable one. Life unfolding cannot be easily quantified.

How would the despair and hopelessness of the "silhouette in the window" be richly illustrated? By what means could the unending grief and sense of devastating losses that subjects experienced be adequately captured? Hence, in order to resolve this dilemma a qualitative method using long interviews was employed.

A detailed discussion of the methodology may be found in the original research (Palmer, 1991) as well as the summation of findings (Palmer, 1997). For the purposes of this report it is noted that all subjects were adult children of alcoholics (ACOAs) who met specific criteria which included age (25-35) and the ability to speak English. A well-tested instrument, CAST, Children of Alcoholics Screening Test (Pilat & Jones, 1984-85), was used to select the sample of ten participants (Chadwick, Bahr, & Albrecht, 1984; McCracken, 1988). Validity and reliability were maintained and methods as well as findings were reviewed by two independent raters whose results were highly consistent with each other and the author. The respondents' life patterns, behaviors, experiences, and current living situations were recorded using the DRM. All four degrees of resiliency were found to be represented among the ten participants. The dynamic features of this instrument were able to capture the processes of survival, transition, and growth. The following are case examples from the subject population who illustrate these features. Comments regarding how practitioners may intervene using this conceptual model are included. The most comprehensive discussion of the DRM model is devoted to Chance, who represents living on the edge in a state of anomic survival and thus presents the greatest challenge for practitioner response. Therein follows a more limited discussion of the model related to other illustrative subjects.

CASE OF CHANCE

This young adult man (all names are pseudonyms) lives in a state of anomic survival much as he had in the home where he grew up. He is the only participant who clearly belongs in this category. Both of his parents were alcoholics. His mother had experienced severe medical problems which were exacerbated by her continual use of alcohol in her efforts to cope. The general home environment was one of omission, i.e., contained little organization or predictable routine, or parental guidance. Violent fights between siblings were frequent. It was survival of the fittest. Chance had found solace through his mother although she was immobilized much of the time. Her presence in the home, the "beacon in the window," had given him a small island of comfort in the midst of violence, uncertainty and the lawlessness of the environment. When she died, Chance was set adrift. Finding no shore, Chance clings to life. He reports abusing alcohol and drugs. His relationships are tenuous having no enduring attachment to anyone. His attachment is to drugs. Chance admits having felt suicidal but never seeking help. He has no support system. In this condition he describes himself as being a "lost soul."

APPLYING FEATURES OF THE DRM

Let the reader assume at the time of intervention, Chance is 14 years old and going through a significant developmental transition. This time is particularly significant as he has just had his 14th birthday. He reports that both his parents "forgot" about this important event. He reports staying out late and experimenting with drugs, including marijuana and alcohol. His brothers, most older, also abuse poly substances and engage in violence in the home and elsewhere as a means of interaction. Chance's home is chaotic. His mother, once a "beacon in the window," has told the children they would have to essentially take care of themselves. She is suffering from serious periodontal disease that has spread systemically. There is no medical insurance, although Father works enough so there is food and shelter. Mother is coping with increasing pain and physical deterioration by increasing her use of alcohol. As she experiences the continued loss of functioning and of her role as a significant nurturing influence in the home, she is becoming immobilized, a silhouette window. Chance's father is coping by staying away from home and increasing his drinking as well. Chance and the family are at a level of anomic survival.

Using the DRM as a guide, immediate response is needed to begin re-balancing the family and re-establishing some consistency in parenting. A strategic area to re-balance the family would be strengthening the existing competence of the parents by providing support. For example, Chance's father provided consistent income but was overwhelmed. Recognizing this contribution is important. Education and support, including identification of strengths, reformation and strengthening of parental boundaries, and development of new parenting responses, could be helpful in achieving a greater sense of cohesiveness and affiliation. Support for the marital relationship may enhance a fragmented partnership. Chance's mother is in need of immediate medical attention, including evaluation for detoxification if necessary and treatment for her dental and physical conditions. Social programs to provide medical care are needed. Because the use of alcohol and other drugs is pervasive, family and individual support and treatment are in order. Alternative ways of managing conflict and defining the competencies of self are needed to reduce or ameliorate the level of violence. The family's relationship with their environment is one of isolation. Avenues for attachment are imperative. For example, Chance loves acting in the theater, the one area where he enjoys some approval and success and where his "acting out" has an appropriate outlet. It is evident that with support and appropriate avenues for expression, such as the theater, Chance may better connect with others and experience a measure of competence and success. His theatrical activities represent an opportunity for further developing his social skills and for learning alternative ways of problem solving. The concepts of "rehearsal" and "audience" are useful in helping Chance learn and "audition" new behaviors and self-expression thus enhancing his attachments to others.

Chance and his family can benefit from re-directing their use of energy to have "sufficient strength to" cope and grow. Chance's mother has little energy for herself, her husband, or her children. The family misses her. Family members use much of their energy engaging in coping behaviors that consume them and create further negative consequences. The children may be motivated for change by the hope of regaining the vital presence of their mother. Family counseling in the home and involving the children in more constructively managing their environment, including daily living, may free up some of their mother's energy and their own so that a more productive level of personal interaction and greater satisfaction could be achieved by all members.

CASE OF ANNA

Anna is one of two respondents who are in transition from anomic survival to regenerative resilience. Her profile is important because her movement toward a degree of resilience was at first negatively affected by the loss of significant others such as her brothers, a favorite aunt, and an admired teacher. As a young child, Anna's brothers protected her and acted as buffers to her mother's alcoholic rages and abuse. She had watched "in horror" as her father raped her mother. Her mother constantly talked of suicide, bringing words close to reality in a bloody episode that almost succeeded. The brothers left home and Anna was then alone to experience and cope with an unending script of violence, sexual abuse, and neglect. When Anna was in the third grade her mother's alcoholism, father's work, and marital conflict contributed to the further alienation and subsequent separation of her parents. Later this separation was made permanent through divorce. Unlike Chance, Anna attempted to get help but "no one listened." Feeling helpless, hopeless, and alone, Anna turned to alcohol and drugs in order to shut out her savage world. At age 15 she left home, marrying a man who also was "violent and a user." When he was sent to prison, Anna began to turn her life around. She sought help again through professional counseling and AA. Anna has been sober for over 4 years and she reports that she is "fifty-per cent satisfied with life where it used to be zero." Her situation illustrates that the use of therapeutic resources can be beneficial in providing support and encouragement when significant others are not available.

CASE OF SAUL

Illustrating regenerative resilience is Saul. Like Anna, Saul also devoted tremendous energy in coping and subsequently mending from the effects of a very violent home. Both of his parents were alcoholic. His father stayed away while his mother, described as "intensely angry," raged within the home. Saul reported his mother lashing out at the children with objects, her shoes, wire coat hangers, anything. He vividly recalled his home "strewn with broken bottles and debris" in the aftermath of his parents' drinking episodes. As the "hero" Saul tried to find a path of acceptance through scholarship, sports, and as a mediator for the family's distress. He turned to alcohol, as did his brothers, in a sense of hopeless pain. Saul "blamed himself" for conditions in the family. In his early 20s he was diagnosed with Bi-Polar Affective Disorder. It was the beginning of 16 hospitalizations. He started medication, therapy, and AA. Saul has been alcohol free for 10 years. He continues therapy, observing, "there is no steady course for a manic-depressive." Saul's long-term marriage with a stable woman in a non-violent home has been healing and affirming of his efforts to develop. His resilience is increasingly evident in his positive outlook about his life and his ability to sustain a measure of quality of life which exceeds survival. His journey exemplifies what it takes to sustain and achieve constructive coping strategies in the face of the constant disruption and challenge of a serious and persistent mental illness.

APPLICATION OF DRM

In contrast to the siblings in Chance's family, siblings in Anna's and Saul's families formed beneficial alliances with one another. Anna reports that her brothers "protected her." Saul describes times when he and his siblings would gather "under the blankets at night" to talk about what was happening in their home. Siblings would "sneak food" to a brother or sister "restricted to the bedroom for days with only bread and water." Both situations illustrate the capacity for attachments and the use of others as benefactors in surviving challenges and adversity. The gathering of siblings, although clandestine and against family rules about "not talking about violence and alcohol," also represents their "will" to transcend their environment. In the process, the children were able in some measure to differentiate "self."

Likewise, in Anna's and Saul's situations the larger social environment had an impact as well. Until recently "rape" was not defined as an illegal act among married adults. The lack of laws and other social institutions addressing a woman's right to her own body regardless of her "attachments" or relationship to others contributes to the continual abuse and sexual assault of women. Practice, then, must consider multiple levels of intervention. "Recognizing resources requires awareness of environmental contexts, sensitivity to cultural differences and openness to a broad range of possibilities" (Miley, 1998, p. 233). Examination of family and personal resources includes: What are the physical and personal abilities and needs of each member? Individual capacities and how each acquires resources to meet his or her or the family's needs. And, how have members coped thus far?

An important area to consider is the family's relationship to their environment. Do they have power in relationship to outside systems or is it overpowered by environmental demands? "Family boundaries can easily become dysfunctional due to the powerlessness stemming from external sources and members societal roles" (Hobbs, Pinderhughes, & Shankar, 1995, p. 53). For example, Saul was experiencing the beginning effects of a severe and persistent mental illness in adolescence. He was labeled as "acting out" and a "behavior problem." His condition went undetected or inappropriately responded to for years. His use of alcohol and drugs was his effort to cope with the pain of his childhood and emerging symptoms.

In a comprehensive study of overwhelmed clients, Hobbs et al. (1995) found that "there is potential for greater clinical success, providing that deficits in the community and neighborhoods and in national policy can be addressed" (p. 24). Thus, social and practitioner response is called for at multiple levels. Recognizing that people and families are "work in process" of survival, repair, or growth, may help practitioners be non-judgmental and more inclusive of larger social systems in their planning and response. Both Anna and Saul showed capacity for attachments and the ability to use resources. A critical factor then becomes how practitioners can advocate, create, and modify the environment to provide greater reciprocity to children and families.

CASE OF ROSE

Rose is one of three subjects who had reached adaptive resilience. Her early memories of being "cuddled on her father's lap and nurtured by her mother" turned into a devastating childhood. Her alcoholic father became progressively violent. Rose and her siblings were "stripped and whipped in front of each other," even when she was twelve years of age. The family was forced to eat broken glass embedded in food that was flung from the refrigerator by her "drunken father." The violence became progressively sadistic. The marriage ended when her father pointed a shotgun at a sibling while ordering her fleeing mother to return home. Her mother soon took the children and left, thus ushering in an era of predictability and relative peace. Rose reported surviving all of these experiences by "escaping through books."

She also had her "secret hiding places" in the home. Her maternal grandparents provided her with their "unconditional love." Their consistent attention gave Rose a thread of humanity. A good student with an inquisitive mind, Rose was able to forge enduring bonds with some of her teachers.

Since divorcing a "quiet alcoholic" and seeking support and therapy, Rose has lived in a "non-violent" supportive environment with another family. She is employed and is able to provide for her physical and emotional needs. She feels safe and secure. These constructive methods of coping enable Rose not only to survive but to achieve a degree of adaptive resilience.

APPLICATION OF DRM

As the reader follows Rose's story of survival in a home with a violent and sadistic father, it would be easy to dismiss the positive capacities and abilities of her parents. Recall that her home was not always this way. To capture the family's transition from Rose's "being cuddled on her father's lap and nurtured by her mother" to being "stripped and whipped" it would be highly desirable to enlist the family as "experts" about its own process of coping and survival. For example, exploring what was different about the early years in the family's development may give the practitioner an idea of the challenges the family was trying to overcome and how they were managing. Such a process may assist the family in its own self awareness of what worked even for a little while (Miley, 1998).

It is critical that the presence of Rose's father not be overlooked as a possible resource to the family. Hobbs et al. (1995) note, "Any serious national intervention must address problems faced by men" (p. 27). "A good place to start is to help them conquer the social stigma and their own sense of uselessness" (Hobbs et al., 1995, p. 145). For example, practitioners may relabel (not excuse) "controlling behavior . . . as an exhausting yet heroic effort to organize the family" (Hobbs et al., 1995, p. 61).

Groups for men in nonclinical settings and without clinical labels, such as "Anger Management Group," may be useful avenues of support and encouragement, and offer alternative ways of problem solving. Utilizing community leaders and peers who have successfully coped may also be helpful to men. An important goal is fostering attachments at multiple levels. Herman (1992) contends that the "core experiences of psychological trauma are disempowerment and disconnection from others" (p. 133). Researchers discovered that in war, the "strongest protection against overwhelming terror was the degree of relatedness between the soldier, his immediate fighting unit, and his leader" (Herman, 1992, p. 25). Given these findings, it follows that social institutions must provide the foundation for meaningful and valued relationships at all levels. Real efforts must be made to help families and partners "re-connect" with each other in nurturing ways. Men must not be excluded from the equation for to do so is to limit the natural resources for individuals, families, and communities.

CASE OF CARMEN

Carmen is one of two subjects who has reached a level of thriving or flourishing resilience. Her journey is traced from a home with an alcoholic father and a mother who was in fragile health much of the time. As in Anna's case, Carmen's brothers provided a measure of support and protection. When they left, she too experienced a spiral into hopelessness and turned to marijuana at age 12 for comfort. While some measure of stability was attained through the regular meals in the home which included open discussions among her siblings (she was the youngest of four), Carmen recalls a life of uncertainty. She was sexually abused by her father's friends. Her father became increasingly "difficult and problematic." Carmen moved rapidly into heavy drug use, reporting "drinking to get drunk." Yet, she was also able to seize opportunities that offered her a way out. Carmen reports that her best friend was involved in church and supported her in connecting with this resource. She "quit doing drugs" and began to flourish in school. She graduated and began attending a private denominational college and was successful in her studies until her emerging homosexual orientation led to expulsion. Carmen turned again to drugs in despair.

Having experienced prejudice and hatred as a child of Cuban refugees and as a lesbian, Carmen felt very much abandoned and alone. She reports feeling "spiritually bankrupted, losing touch with God." Once again, seeing potential avenues of renewal through the graduation of a friend from college, Carmen returned to her studies at a different institution. She was able to obtain intensive therapy and is now sober. Her spiritual life, once empty, is now "flourishing" with her integration of the church as a constant resource. Carmen has almost completed a college degree and she supports herself through the use of her linguistic skills in Spanish to help others who are not bi-lingual. Her sense of coherence about life, the valuing of herself, her orientation and heritage are evident. In a long-term stable relationship Carmen continues to flourish. As a woman who is Hispanic and lesbian, Carmen represents survival not only within an alcoholic home, but also with the larger context of society.

APPLICATION OF DRM

Carmen's history represents, on a larger scale, the need to have "justice-based clinical work" that contributes to community building (Hobbs et al.,

1995, p. 144). To do so, a practitioner must sharpen one's "knowledge about the realities of racism and classism, and their interplay including the particulars of class structure and the effects of poverty" (Lee, 1994, p. 22). Carmen's parents fled Cuba to escape political terrorism. "Those who work with war survivors must recognize the family's efforts to maintaining cohesion in the face of catastrophic losses, including loss of one's culture and community" (Webb, 1991, p. 108). Lum (1999) advises that "people of color have internal and external values that are a part of one's being, and existence as a cultural and ethnic person" (p. 36). Practice response must consider the tremendous strength and courage that Carmen's family has as natural resources for themselves and their community.

The issue of sexual orientation contributes to the tension and disconnection between Carmen and her environments. Safety is of critical importance and requires attention to not only her physical safety but also protection from the "realities of power" in social situations (Herman, 1992, p. 171). Like the previous case illustrations, community and group work is a viable option even though not the "preferred" strategy (Hobbs et al., 1995, p. 86). Groups may be helpful "when parents are functionally absent due to drug abuse or other debilitating circumstances" (Hobbs et al., 1995, p. 133). Groups can support personal and collective power, enhance solidarity as protection against terror and despair, provide a sense of belonging in the face of social oppression and isolation, create opportunities for people to bear witness, and affirm where shame and stigmatization reside (Herman, 1991). Cross-systems approaches utilizing a solution-focused and strengths perspective are particularly important for people who have been alienated (DeJong & Miller, 1995). Groups and community efforts can make significant contributions in the form of energy and services for regeneration, repair, growth, and change. In order to flourish and thrive, children and their families must significantly exceed the minimum requirements for survival and safety. They must have greater reserves of energy than beyond that required for survival. Reciprocity, therefore, must often begin with social institutions and the larger environment. Practitioners can be instrumental in transforming social institutions and communities into avenues that fuel and nurture families.

In review, by far the vast majority of these ACOAs are functioning better than expected. Half of the 10 respondents are in the higher functioning categories of adaptive resilience (three) and flourishing resilience (two) (Table 1). One subject is in transition to adaptive resilience. Thus, at least 60 percent of the ACOAs have demonstrated sustained periods of stability and balance, with regular use of competencies and coping strategies. These individuals are experiencing sustained reciprocity with the external environments of home and elsewhere. Individuals who are thriving have also developed a sense of meaning to their lives that transcends daily living. Antonovsky

TABLE 1. Subject Functioning in Terms of Resiliency

SUBJECT NAME	TYPE OF RESILIENCY	TRANSITION TO TYPE OF RESILIENCY
CHANCE	Anomic Survival	
ANNA		Transition to Regenerative Resiliency
MAC		Transition to Regenerative Resiliency
SAUL	Regenerative Resiliency	
MARY		Transition to Adaptive Resiliency
ROSE	Adaptive Resiliency	
JOE	Adaptive Resiliency	
SAM	Adaptive Resiliency	
CARMEN	Flourishing Resiliency	
LUCY	Flourishing Resiliency	

(1985) identified the sense of coherence about life and self as essential to thriving. Flach (1988) found the spiritual dimension is an important resource for resilient individuals.

LESSON FIVE: IMPLICATIONS FOR PRACTICE

The Differential Resiliency Model presents a new language that attempts to capture life-in-process in non-pathological terms. Referring to children and youth as "at-risk," or impoverished, or by other professional or social labels, "burdens them with the expectation that they will fail" to paraphrase Butler (1997, p. 25). Social workers and other helping professionals, community leaders, and other citizens concerned with children may find the DRM a useful model for better understanding the process of survival and growth. Practitioners may use the DRM in combination with other measures such as the CAST to produce information about the presence and degrees of resilience so that they can initiate or coordinate more timely and appropriate responses that complement the efforts of children and their families to survive and grow. "Attention to only the negative symptomatic aspects of the families of addicted people leads to stereotyping and denying the many resources and coping strategies of these families" (Anderson, 1994, p. 680). This preposition need not be restricted to families who are struggling with alcohol and substance abuse. One may apply the central premise of an ethic of non-pathology across cultures and communities. For example, the Spanish language has no verb that means "to cope" but rather the expression *tener suficiente fuerza para* (to have sufficient strength to) clarifies the essence of this concept (Lee, 1994, p. 80). Manning (1997) postulates that as moral citizens, social workers should be aware "of the underlying distribution of power through theoretical models" (p. 228). For example, an unexpected finding from many of the respondents was the consistent indication of their efforts to reach out for help in some way to others, including child welfare workers, only to have their efforts ignored, misinterpreted, or misdiagnosed because of their outward behavior. This finding received recent support from another study (Freeman & Dyer, 1993) that concluded that "the DSM-III-R diagnoses for youngsters are individually focused; consequently, the diagnoses do not consider the effects of the neighborhood and family risk factors such as substance abuse, negative modeling of problem-solving skills, and violence" (p. 429). Tracy (1994) and Fraser (1996) made similar observations in their examinations of interventions with multi-problem youths. The continued focus on pathology and even the subtle influence of identifying children "at-risk" may contribute to the lack of sensitive appreciation for an individual's or family's efforts to cope or find sufficient strength to manage adversity and the challenges of daily living.

LESSON SIX: WHAT WE CAN LEARN FROM SURVIVORS AND THRIVERS

We can learn much from those who live daily with incredible adversity. DesPres (1977) reflects on life in the death camps, the Holocaust, "My subject is survival, the capacity of men and women to live beneath the pressure of protracted crisis, to sustain terrible damage in mind and body, and yet, be there, sane, alive, still human" (p. v). The lessons learned from the survivors and thrivers in this study are highlighted as follows.

Factors Negatively Impacting Coping

- Loss of significant others in early life
- Other losses such as health, or medical or financial support
- No sources of support for personal validation or self-worth
- Inability to elicit help from others or find others who respond appropriately

- Lack of skills required to elicit positive responses from the environment
- Energy required for survival leaves little energy for repair or growth
- The younger the age of trauma, the greater the severity of impacts particularly on human attachments

Resources Positively Impacting Coping

- Siblings who offer support and/or protection
- Ability to develop creative ways to survive, such as finding secret hiding places
- Ability to connect with the environment through means such as domestic or work activities, church, and other socially organized institutions
- Social attachments to well functioning adults or peers
- The "will" to have something better than in the past
- Ability to reframe one's experiences into a useful lesson
- Ability to seek and make use of professional or self-help therapeutic interventions
- Ability to assess reality for what it is and have some concept of "self" as a valuable identity

LESSON SEVEN: IMPLICATION FOR A COLLECTIVE RESPONSE

Survivors should be viewed in the context in which their struggle takes place. At one level is the family, kinship system, and significant others. At another level is the larger social context. The latter also exerts a significant influence on the capacity of our children to thrive. For example, "the black family in its variations has provided the structure and support for its members to overcome tremendous economic, political, and social obstacles" (Crawley, 1988, p. 416). In another perspective Germain (1991) has described institutional and social oppression as "social pollutions." These include the annihilation of culture as a coping mechanism. One's home and family constitute a culture and should thus be approached has having value. Our response calls for collective action.

"People who are struggling to survive generally live in communities that are struggling for economic survival" (Lee, 1994, p. 265). Therein lies a link between the subject of survival and poverty. Manning (1997) highlighted the idea that "moral citizenship is transformational, changing the structures of oppression to structures more congruent with social work values" (p. 224). It is not just practitioners, however, who have a moral obligation. It is all of us. Most apparent from this study is the finding that human relatedness, that is, the capacity to form attachments, be it with a grandparent baking cookies, a youth group in a church, or the kin network of persons, offers a significant measure of support and reciprocity, while providing energy for growth and thriving.

This research is only one small study, but hopefully it contributes to a new conceptual framework that may energize our own resources to engage others. If we re-define pathology into competencies and creative responses to protracted crisis, we could stimulate thought about our obligations to others. This model is presented to: (a) create new ways of embracing the variations of human expression, human condition, and human efforts to survive, grow, and thrive, and (b) provide a practical means of matching and/or developing community and national resources for families and children. Hopefully this will enhance our efforts to help others develop their personal growth and resilience in the face of life's inevitable adversities.

EPILOGUE

There is a rich tapestry of history, a tapestry whose stories are woven in the souls of its makers. If we listen, if we open our ears to their voices, if we see their lives unfolding, we have much to learn. Chance, his family, and others need not end up as statistics. We must not settle for *survival* or a *good enough* quality of life. It is a moral imperative that the only acceptable standard of professional and social response is one of enabling children and their families to grow and thrive. We must never be content to live with a single silhouette in the window. These are the lessons learned from adversity. Now is our turn to apply them.

BIBLIOGRAPHY

Anderson, S. (1994). A critical analysis of the concept of codependency. *Social Work, 39* (6), 671-685.

Anthony, E.J., & Cohler, B.J. (Eds.). (1987). *The invulnerable child.* New York: The Guilford Press.

Anthony, E.J. (1987). Risk, vulnerability, and resilience: An overview. In E.J. Anthony & B.J. Cohler (Eds.). *The invulnerable child* (pp. 3-48). New York: The Guilford Press.

Antonovsky, A. (1985). *Health, stress, and coping.* SF: Jossey-Bass.

Butler, K. (1997, March/April). The anatomy of resilience. *Family Therapy Networker*, 22-31.

Chadwick, B.A., Bahr, H.M., & Albrecht, S.L. (1984). *Social science research methods*. Englewood Cliffs, New Jersey: Prentice-Hall, Inc.

Cowen, E.L. & Work, W. (1988). Resilient children, psychological wellness, and primary prevention. *American Journal of Community Psychiatry, 16 (4)*, 591-607.

Crawley, B. (1988, October). Black Families in a Neo-Conservative era. *Family Relations 37, (4)*, 419-515.

De Jong, P., & Miller, S. (1995). How to interview for client strengths. *Social Work 40* (5), 729-736.

DesPres, T. (1977). *The survivor: Anatomy of life in the death camps*. NY: Pocket Books.

El-Guebaly, N. & Offord, D.R. (1977, April). The offspring of alcoholics: A critical review. *American Journal of Psychiatry, 134 (4)*, 357-364.

Felsman, J.K., & Vaillant, G.E. (1987). Resilient children as adults: A 40-year study. In E.J. Anthony & B.J. Cohler (Eds.). *The invulnerable child* (pp. 289-313). New York: The Guilford Press.

Flach, F. (1988). *Resilience: Discovering a new strength at times of stress*. New York: Fawcett Columbine.

Fraser, M. (1966). Aggressive behavior in childhood and early adolescence: An ecological-developmental perspective on youth violence. *Social Work 41, (4)*, 347-361.

Germain, C. (1991). *Human behavior and the social environment*. NY: Columbia University Press.

Herman, J. (1992). *Truama and recovery: The aftermath of violence from domestic abuse and political terror*. New York: Basic Books.

Hopps, J., Pinderhughes, E., Shankar, R. (1995). *The power to care: Clinical practice effectiveness with overwhelmed clients*. New York: The Free Press.

Lee, J. (1994). *The empowerment approach to social work practice*. NY: Columbia University Press.

Lum, D. (1999). *Culturally competent practice: A framework for growth and action*. Pacific Grove, CA: Brooks/Cole.

Manning, S. (1997). The social worker as moral citizen: Ethics in action. *Social Work 42, (3)*, 223-230.

Miley, K., O'Melia, M., & DuBois, B. (1998). *Generalist social work practice: An empowering approach*. Boston: Allyn & Bacon.

McCracken, G. (1988). *The long interview*. Newbury Park: Sage.

Murphy, L.B., & Moriarty, A.E. (1976). *Vulnerability coping and growth: From infancy to adolescence*. London: Yale University Press.

Palmer, N. (1991). Exploring resiliency in adult children of alcoholics. Doctoral Dissertation. University of Kansas.

Palmer, N. (1997, August) Resilience in adult children of alcoholics: A nonpathological approach to social work practice. *Health and Social Work (22), (3)*, 201-209.

Parker, D.A., & Harford, T.C. (1988). Alcohol-related, marital disruption and depressive symptoms among adult children of alcohol abusers in the United States. *Journal of Studies on Alcohol, 49, (4)*, 306-31.

Pearsall, P. (1998). *The heart's code: Tapping the wisdom and power of heart energy*. NY: Broadway Books.

Pilat, J.M. & Jones, J.W. (1984/85). Identification of children of alcoholics: Two empirical studies. *Alcohol Health and Research World*, (Winter) 27-36.

Saleebey, D. (1996). The strengths perspective in social work practice: Extensions and cautions. *Social Work, 41 (3)*, 296-305.

Tracy, E. (1994). Maternal substance abuse: Protecting the child, preserving the family. *Social Work 39, (5)*, 534-539.

Webb, N. (1991). *Play therapy with children in crisis: A casebook for practitioners*. New York: Guilford Press.

Weick, A. (1983) Issues in overturning a medical model of social work practice. *Social Work 28*, *(6)*, 467-471.

Zastrow, C.D., Kirst-Ashmen, K. (1990). *Understanding human behavior and the social environment*. Chicago: Nelson-Hall Publishers.

Ecumenical Housing: Providing Housing and Services

Christopher Krehmeyer
Peter W. Salsich, Jr.
Cathryne L. Schmitz

SUMMARY. Over the last two decades child and family poverty has increased while resources for families at risk have decreased. Families in large urban areas, faced with increasing poverty and isolation, are at very high risk. Economic, and often racial, isolation leaves these families struggling amidst inadequate resources as they attempt to move their children into a position of strength. Without adequate, stable, safe housing families cannot meet their most basic needs. Beyond housing, families need access to the resources and services which help them gain the personal and job skills needed to gain economic self-sufficiency. This article reviews the development of one agency's work to provide the housing and support services low income single mothers need to help them move to a position of self-sufficiency. *[Article copies available for a fee from The Haworth Document Delivery Service: 1-800-342-9678. E-mail address: getinfo@haworthpressinc.com <Website: http://www.haworthpressinc.com>]*

KEYWORDS. Low income housing, poverty, self-sufficiency, economic isolation

---

Christopher Krehmeyer is Executive Director, Ecumenical Housing, Production Corporation, Saint Louis, MO.

Peter W. Salsich, Jr., is McDonnell Professor of Justice in American Society School of Law, Saint Louis University.

Cathryne L. Schmitz, ACSW, PhD, is affiliated with the Graduate School of Social Work, University of Denver.

[Haworth co-indexing entry note]: "Ecumenical Housing: Providing Housing and Services." Krehmeyer, Christopher, Peter W. Salsich, Jr., and Cathryne L. Schmitz. Co-published simultaneously in *Social Thought* (The Haworth Pastoral Press, an imprint of The Haworth Press, Inc.) Vol. 19, No. 2, 1999, pp. 89-102; and: *Raising Our Children Out of Poverty* (ed: John J. Stretch et al.) The Haworth Pastoral Press, an imprint of The Haworth Press, Inc., 1999, pp. 89-102. Single or multiple copies of this article are available for a fee from The Haworth Document Delivery Service [1-800-342-9678, 9:00 a.m. - 5:00 p.m. (EST). E-mail address: getinfo@haworthpressinc.com].

Poverty is "one of America's more enduring social problems" (Scarpetti & Cylke, 1995). More than a fifth (20.5%) of America's children live in poverty. For African American children the number is even higher–39.9% (Children's Defense Fund [CDF], 1998). Children in female-headed single parent families are at the highest risk. Because of gender inequality and the low income of women, the biggest risk facing female-headed households is poverty (Schmitz, 1995). At a poverty rate of 49.3%, female headed single parent families are the country's poorest demographic group, with the greatest risk among Hispanic and African American families (CDF, 1998).

The recurrent debate over welfare reform has negatively impacted the most vulnerable. This has disproportionately included single parent families and children (Bryner, 1998). Lacking stability and resources, two fifths (42%) of women who leave welfare often return within the first two years (Harris, 1996). The welfare debate and current changes go beyond the change from AFDC to Temporary Assistance for Needy Families (TANF). The debates and budget cuts include the basic safety net surrounding our poorest and most vulnerable, primarily children. Budget cutting policies which began in the 1980s resulted in cuts in public housing, Aid for Families with Dependent Children (AFDC), food stamps, and Medicaid (CDF, 1992). Conditions have worsened since the 1995 Republican "Contract with America" intensified budget cuts (Sanger, 1995) in programs that heavily impact single parent families (Gray, 1995).

National welfare policy and national housing policy are intertwined in their impact on family self-sufficiency (Salsich, 1997). American cities are facing a housing crisis (Schwartz, Bartlet, Ferlauto, & Hoffman, 1992). Public housing policies creating large projects have isolated families in inferior neighborhoods (Koebel, 1997), aggravating the problems. The number of very low income families (50 percent or less of area median income) who are paying more than 50 percent of their income for rent has reached a record 5.3 million in the United States (U.S. Dept., 1998). Single-parent female-headed families, congregated in metropolitan areas, struggle with economic (Jargowsky & Wilson, 1997) and social structures which limit the potential for economic growth.

Programs designed to help families move from TANF to self-sufficiency must recognize and address the multiple needs of low income, primarily female-headed single parent families. Families without adequate housing do not have the resources to participate in employment or even job training. In order for families to gain the skills and knowledge needed, families must have financial and social supports (Schmitz, 1995) as well as stable, affordable housing (Salsich, 1997). This article provides a review of the development and expansion of a non-profit scattered site housing program designed to address the housing, resource, and social needs of low income, primarily single parent female-headed single parent households.

Ecumenical Housing Production Corporation (EHPC) is a not for profit corporation which constructs and rehabilitates housing for low income families. The housing consists of single family homes located in scattered sites throughout municipalities and neighborhoods primarily in St. Louis County. As of April 1998, EHPC owns and operates over 180 homes and houses well over 750 individuals including more than 500 children. From its inception in 1980, EHPC has endeavored to create an environment that fosters personal growth for the entire family. EHPC describes its management style as "pastoral," meaning that it gives equal emphasis to the needs of its resident families ("soft" management) as it does to the needs of its property ("hard" management). An ambitious supportive services program is aimed at strengthening families, improving parenting, and encouraging children's educational, emotional and psychological growth. In addition, EHPC helps heads of household empower themselves, improve their job skills and further their education in order to realize their fullest potential.

The homes produced by EHPC blend into established neighborhoods, and often are some of the most attractive homes on a block. Typically, tenants have average yearly incomes under $11,000. Ninety-seven percent of EHPC's families are headed by women in their thirties, with three children, who qualify to participate in the federal Section 8 rental assistance program. More than one-third of the families who have lived in EHPC's units have been able to move from the welfare rolls into the economic and housing mainstream. Those who remain in EHPC properties become stabilized and experience individual growth, while their children live in safe, positive environments where they are able to make substantial progress in decent schools.

CREATION OF EHPC

EHPC was born out of a serious public controversy over subsidized housing in St. Louis County. In the late 1970s, St. Louis County had an expanding population of nearly 1 million people and was experiencing significant job growth. By contrast, jobs and living conditions in the city of St. Louis, where the population hovered around 400,000, were declining (East-West Gateway, 1996).

A major school desegregation lawsuit in St. Louis was settled in 1980 by a consent decree that established a voluntary inter-district busing program (*Liddell v. Board of Education*, 1980). One element of the consent decree was a requirement that a plan be developed for using federal housing subsidies to help create integrated neighborhoods and thus eventually alleviate the need for the inter-district busing program (*Liddell v. Board of Education* consent decree, § 12.d). The St. Louis area regional planning agency, East-West Gateway Co-ordinating Council, had developed a draft plan for regional fair share housing, but had been unsuccessful in persuading member local governments to implement the plan (East-West Gateway, 1972). Meanwhile, an acrimonious public controversy broke out between St. Louis County government officials and the local office of the Department of Housing and Urban Development (HUD) over HUD's desire to provide federal housing subsidies for a proposed low income family apartment complex in Earth City, an unincorporated area along the Missouri River in the northwest corner of St. Louis County that was being developed as an office and light industrial park.

The confluence of these three events: (a) the fair housing element of the school consent decree, (b) the failure of the East-West Gateway regional housing plan, and (c) the public controversy over Earth City housing caused individuals who were active in local religious organizations as well as civic and social action organizations to begin a series of informal meetings over breakfast in 1979 at a popular meeting place in St. Louis County. Unsuccessful efforts to mediate a settlement of the HUD-St. Louis County housing dispute led to a decision to incorporate as a Missouri not-for-profit corporation and become a housing developer in St. Louis County. The name, Ecumenical Housing Development Corporation, was chosen to emphasize three features agreed to by the founders of EHPC: (a) an ecumenical Judeo-Christian philosophy of pastoral stewardship, (b) an emphasis on housing, and (c) a desire to own and manage the housing that was to be developed. EHPC's stated objectives as it began operations were threefold: (a) make additional housing available for qualifying low income families; (b) demonstrate that rental housing for low and moderate income families can be a community asset and a positive contribution to neighborhoods in suburban St. Louis County; and (c) create a model of church, industry, and government working together to address a critical community and human problem (Gottman, 1980).

EHPC was incorporated out of a sense of frustration that little or no effort was being made in suburban St. Louis to offer housing for low income families in integrated environments. Despite its growth and relative affluence, St. Louis County had a serious and growing need for more affordable housing. The vacancy rate for all size and price rental units in St. Louis County was 2.1%, a vacancy rate largely caused by the "turnover," not by available units. The situation was particularly critical for low and moderate income families who needed more than one or two bedrooms. In August 1980, over 4500 families were on a waiting list maintained by the St. Louis County Housing Authority for public or assisted housing. Twenty percent of those families needed three bedroom units, but only thirteen percent of the approximately 6100 assisted housing units in St. Louis County had three or more bedrooms (Gottman, 1980). Over 20,000 families (8.2%) had incomes of less than $5,000. Median family incomes were under $10,000 in twenty-eight of the ninety-two municipalities in St. Louis County. The average price of a three bedroom home in St. Louis County in 1979 was $53,000. Because low income families could not afford home ownership, these families competed for and doubled up in available rental units costing 30-50% of their monthly family income (Tobin as cited in Gottman, 1980).

The founders of EHPC, a group of architects, contractors, lawyers, and community and religious leaders, sought to fill that gap by acquiring and rehabilitating existing single family homes in deteriorated condition that were scattered throughout the county. The hope was that properties could be purchased cheaply, and that some foreclosed properties might even be donated. The founders believed that some homes could be renovated with volunteer labor drawn from supportive civic and church groups. EHPC would select families to lease the homes. Section 8 assistance would pay the bulk of the rent.

EHPC chose to focus its efforts in the inner ring suburbs of St. Louis County for three reasons. First, many not-for-profits and for-profit housing developers were active in the City of St. Louis at that time, but none were active in St. Louis County. Second, board members wanted to support efforts to provide integrated, mixed-income housing in the suburbs. Finally, board members believed that the less crowded, predominately single family settings of the suburbs offered a better environment for family-oriented housing.

EHPC's founders and early Board of Directors recognized that the environment in which families live has a tremendous impact on their ability to move forward in their lives economically and psychologically. This belief is reiterated by Lawson and Wilson (1995).

> The social and political isolation of the poor has become more marked in the 1980's and 1990's. In the United States, poverty has become more urban, more concentrated, and more firmly implanted in inner-city neighborhoods in large metropolises, particularly in older industrial cities with immense and highly segregated numbers of blacks and Hispanics. Even the most pessimistic observers of urban life in America during the ghetto riots of the 1960's hardly anticipated the massive breakdown of social institutions in these neighborhoods and the severity of the problems of joblessness, family disruptions, teenage pregnancy, failing schools, and crime and drugs that now involve many of those who live in the inner city. (p. 694)

Therefore, the EHPC Board focused on building a comprehensive program in the inner ring suburbs rather than the central city.

Once in a stable environment, families served by EHPC could focus those areas of their lives that would lead to economic independence, improved family life, and enhanced community living. In retrospect, the concept seems very simple. It was the implementation that proved difficult.

The board agreed to operate and oversee the acquisition, development and management functions until funds could be raised to hire a professional staff. Board members provided both policy direction and hands-on expertise.

Lynn Broeder, EHPC's initial staff consultant and first executive director who served from 1980 until 1993, recruited many of the persons who comprised the first board. EHPC began at a time when interest rates were in the high double digits. Because of its desire to avoid increasing the concentration of subsidized housing in impacted areas, EHPC concentrated its early efforts in stable inner ring suburbs in the central and southern parts of St. Louis County. The search for a place to start that would demonstrate the potential for subsidized family housing in stable suburban neighborhoods took approximately one and one half years, primarily because of the relatively higher costs for housing in such neighborhoods. On May 27, 1981, EHPC closed on the purchase of a duplex in Richmond Heights, a stable middle class suburb bordering the south-central portion of the City of St. Louis (Ecumenical Housing [EHPC], 1981).

PASTORAL MANAGEMENT: A BLEND OF "HARD" AND "SOFT" MANAGEMENT

From the beginning, EHPC concentrated on working with families with children. EHPC's first two property managers were Roman Catholic nuns who brought a concern for, and background in, providing counseling and social services to resident families. In addition to helping families understand and discharge their responsibilities for paying rent on time and keeping their homes neat and clean, EHPC property managers provided equipment for families to care for their yards, and encouraged adult members to register to vote and become involved in neighborhood activities.

A grant from the United States bishops' Campaign for Human Development in the 1980s enabled EHPC to help tenants aspire to become community leaders. In the words of former property manager, Sr. Mary Ann Nestel, CSJ, "When our folks come to us their self-confidence is (tiny). They've been knocked down and stepped on. The opportunity to open the door for them is really exciting" (Kenny, 1988).

Property managers are responsible for traditional real estate management services, as well as the delivery of personalized tenant assistance. EHPC's family assistance program provides educational, job training, and financial management assistance, including helping with job applications, finding day care or transportation, or providing counseling when family crises occur. If a tenant's needs go beyond the experience and capability of the property manager, EHPC offers referrals to other community social service resources.

Combining traditional real estate management with personal family assistance is a complex and challenging task. EHPC's Property Management Committee in 1987 described the family assistance part of its management program as an art.

> All of our tenants need EHPC's help–or they wouldn't be here. There's a wide variation in their individual needs–some need just a little help to rebuild their lives and work their way out of poverty. Others, while doing their best for themselves and their families, will never be self supporting. . . . [T]his doesn't mean that they won't have far better lives because of our efforts. And by having their children in the better schools of EHPC neighborhoods we do, in the long run, help to break the cycle of poverty and dependence. (EHPC, p. 1, 1987)

Because of the long waiting lists for public and subsidized housing in both St. Louis City and County, EHPC has had from its inception the mixed blessing of an extraordinarily strong demand for its houses. As a result EHPC has been able to focus its admission policies on selecting motivated tenants who accept EHPC's philosophy of striving for self sufficiency (EHPC, 1987). However, EHPC staff also have to face the anguish of families who are told there is no room for them.

In the selection process, EHPC staff and board members early on faced the question of whether to require applicants to be employed or in school as a condition for selection as tenants. In recommending against such requirements, the Property Management Committee stated:

> This sounds like a simple issue–but becomes quite complex. For one thing, as part of our mission we deliberately seek out families with children. Many of them are single-parent families with small children. We don't think mothers with young children should be forced to leave the home.
>
> There are other problems with employment. Many of the entry level jobs are only part time, minimum wage jobs. The hiring companies . . . don't have to pay any fringe benefits. . . . Unfortunately, as soon as one of our tenants takes one of these jobs . . . they lose their medicaid health benefits for the whole family. (EHPC, p. 3, 1987)

A management program featuring regular personal contact with tenants to encourage and enable them to maximize their potential as families and as individuals is labor intensive and expensive. EHPC estimates that it costs approximately $200 per unit per month to provide personal family enablement programs. That cost is in addition to the $450 per unit per month needed to amortize loans, maintain property, and pay core staff (EHPC, 1997). Funding for the "soft" management family support efforts must come from sources outside the rental stream and traditional housing assistance programs. EHPC has raised this money primarily from religious and charitable organizations. As the number of units increases, the amount that must be raised annually increases correspondingly.

SOCIAL SERVICE PROGRAM EXPANSION

The social service programs at EHPC have expanded greatly since the early 1980s. In the beginning, family service programs were limited primarily to those that could be provided by the property managers. But EHPC's staff and board recognized over time that, in order for its families to be successful, a broader range of services had to be provided.

In late 1992 funding was secured from the Housing Resource Commission of St. Louis County to begin the Partners in Self-Sufficiency Program (PSS). PSS is a program that provides scholarships for career education and employment training, as well as day care and transportation to help tenants reach self-sufficiency. In addition to this direct monetary support, monthly group meetings and regular mail and phone contact enable EHPC staff and participating residents to offer and receive encouragement, motivation, and support. Personal goals, obstacles encountered, and losses suffered are discussed in the group meetings. Residents often receive positive feedback and reinforcement in these sessions (Schmitz, 1997, p. 4). The PSS has had extraordinary success in moving almost 70% of its participants from welfare to work, by combining resources and a humanistic approach to addressing real life issues.

Sex education classes for mothers and daughters have been added to EHPC services, as have money management and job interview counseling programs. EHPC also has developed educational enrichment programs that allow parents and children to spend time together while participating in art projects and story telling, or while visiting the science and art museum.

EHPC also has seasonal programs that have evolved during its existence. Holiday Friends is a program that provides gifts and Christmas trimmings for members of every tenant family so that they can have an enjoyable holiday season. The Back-to-School Program provides back to school supplies to over 200 children every year. Also, an annual family picnic is a social gathering for tenant families, staff and board members.

Perhaps the program that best demonstrates EHPC's commitment to families and children is the summer camp, which has become a mainstay of the organization. By securing camp scholarships, EHPC provides an opportunity for children between the ages of 6 and 16 to attend overnight camp for a week. Not only is this fun, but it offers an enriching learning experience for the children. It also provides a respite for single mothers who are burdened with heavy responsibilities, which is sorely needed in families that all too often have had a series of crises and setbacks. Nearly 100 children participate in this program every year.

In addition, The Youth Mentor Program was started in 1997, focusing on teenagers living in EHPC homes in the hopes of positioning them for success. Success might be college, vocational school or some other type of meaningful endeavor. Field trips to colleges in Missouri and Illinois have occurred and tutoring and mentoring are available.

Finally, the State of Missouri recently awarded EHPC a "Case Management" grant to provide services to 60 current welfare recipients living in EHPC homes. This welfare-to-work project is the latest evolution in service delivery for EHPC. While the organization has great reservations about the new federal law and the state's implementation of that law, it decided to cooperate with state officials in creating a program to move TANF recipients to work within the short time frame of the law. A tight structure of training, job readiness and employment search was created. EHPC is working with both job training organizations and employers to ensure that participating EHPC families will be able to secure jobs and avoid any potential negative consequences.

With its growing awareness of the difficulties of reversing the effects of years of abuse, poor education and poverty, EHPC's board and staff realized the need to expand its program. The focus now is on the entire family unit and "success" now is seen as a series of small interlocking steps involving two generations. EHPC operates with a yearly budget of more than $2 million. Currently, there are 23 paid staff persons and more than 1,000 active volunteers, including tenants, who work in a variety of positions.

PROGRAM IMPACT ON CHILDREN AND POVERTY

EHPC has engaged in ongoing evaluation by outside evaluators to determine the impact that EHPC's housing and related services programs have on the families. Preliminary results indicate that the impact is extremely positive. Early evaluation (Kelly, 1994) found that EHPC's combination of a stable housing environment and comprehensive "soft management" services can add considerable economic value to the lives of its resident families, as well as to society in general. In addition to the value families obtain by becoming self sufficient, the leveraging effect on government assistance savings is staggering. Using a present value analysis, Kelly estimated that if just 25% of EHPC's 150 single parent families in 1994 broke the cycle of poverty, became self sufficient, and remained so until all children reached the age of 18, the amount of public funds (pre-TANF) that would be saved because these families remained off welfare would exceed $50 million (Kelly, 1994, p. 14).

Subsequent evaluation (Schmitz, 1997) of families living in EHPC housing and participating in the Partners in Self-Sufficiency Program provides evidence of continued program success. Women participating in the program exhibit a dramatic decrease in reliance on AFDC/TANF. Of the 37 women in the program for 1996/97, 16 (43%) were receiving AFDC when they entered the Program. By 1998 only 3 (8%) women were receiving TANF; one because of disability. The vast majority (92%) of the women were employed full or part time compared to 51% at entry. The research indicates that the women are able to maintain their employment because they live in stable, safe housing connected to the resources and supports needed to gain personal and job related skills.

The combination of stable, safe and adequate scattered site housing with resources and support moves the women forward. The comments of the women provide a qualitative context on the program components which have assisted the women.

- I like the fact that the house is blended in with people who are working class, that encourages me. Because I was on welfare when I first started renting. And now just living in the area that I live in helped encourage me which I finished school to do better. Because people around me were working and had that education. So, just being in that environment was encouraging.
- It is a big jump from the city to the county and then the school districts are different. . . . I mean it makes you just work harder to get it. You know, you're like, how can you possibly sit at home and do nothing. I've got to get this and that and do this.
- You do have to get adjusted to it. You see the other people in the neighborhood do it and you got to keep up (Schmitz, 1997, p. 11).

The program has engaged and impacted the children and youth as well.

- It [the children's activities] just gives them something to look forward to. I mean not only just going out on field trips. I mean they just want to, like participate. And my daughters are even older. And most teenagers want to stop going. And I have two teenagers and they still want to (Schmitz, p. 16).

The move precipitated growth for the women and the children. They increased their belief in their own ability to change. The women have moved forward with their education and training through structured support and thoughtful provision of resources.

Kelly (1994) describes the EHPC model as "community based, family oriented, economic development. . . . EHPC is much more than housing. It is the use of housing to make individuals and their families productive citizens" (p. 2).

> In human terms, the value of a home cannot be over estimated. With a home comes shelter from the natural and unnatural elements, drugs, crime and violence. A home also provides a safe place to care for children; a clean, safe place to prepare nutritious meal; a place where people are protected from accidents and infectious diseases; a place to store and maintain clothing; a quiet place to study and plan; and an address to receive information and benefits. (Kelly, 1994, pp. 2, 4)

PROGRAM RESULTS

EHPC began by developing quality scattered site housing. It has grown into a holistic housing network which moves low income families from concentrated poverty to mixed income neighborhoods. This move broadens the horizons of the women as well as the children. Over the years EHPC's services have expanded to meet the multiple needs of the families–support, education, training.

The staff continually refines and changes the program in response to the needs of the families. The lessons learned provide a model for developing similar programs in other localities. Housing, support, and resources underlie the need to empower the most vulnerable families to move toward self-sufficiency. EHPC's model of housing with resources and supports identifies the basic building blocks for successful empowerment of low income women and children.

The intangibles of self esteem and self confidence grow immeasurably from the support and guidance of EHPC programs and staff. Success is measured in a series of small interlocking steps that build upon themselves. EHPC and its unique service delivery method provide, in essence, two critical assets to its families: hope and opportunity. Hope that there is a better life for everyone in the family, particularly the children. Opportunity, realistic opportunities to achieve the dreams and goals to which these families strive.

CONCLUSION

In reflecting on EHPC's almost 20 years of existence, one is left with ambivalent feelings. On one hand, EHPC can be proud of its ability to provide good quality housing in safe and stable neighborhoods to 180 families, including over 500 children. EHPC's program clearly has made a significant difference in their lives. However, when this accomplishment is measured against the fact that approximately 38,000 such families were seeking decent housing in metropolitan St. Louis (and 5.3 million families nationwide) in 1995, one realizes that EHPC's success is a drop in the proverbial bucket. In addition, the energy expended in raising the additional $200 per unit per month to provide the services package is considerable. A way must be found to leverage the EHPC model.

Two approaches are being pursued by EHPC. The first one involves a public-private partnership organized by EHPC to combine resources and revitalize an entire neighborhood, Castlepoint, in north St. Louis County. Approximately 5000 people reside in Castlepoint, a predominantly African-American community. While average household income in 1990 was $30,820, about 14% earned less than $10,000. EHPC has joined with St. Louis County government, The Monsanto Fund, not-for-profit service providers, and local neighborhood organizations to prepare a revitalization plan. This expansion of service delivery area, while leveraging EHPC's program, will stretch the limits of EHPC's resources.

A second leveraging effort is the creation of a management company that would extend the EHPC management program to units supported by a capital partner that raises money to invest in low income housing tax credit (LIHTC) supported housing developments. Should a contract be negotiated, EHPC's inventory of housing units receiving its services would double within one year. EHPC's board approved the management plan concept in August 1998. Under the plan, a new asset and property management organization will be created by EHPC with the following objectives: (a) integrate support service delivery in its operation on a day-to-day basis, (b) achieve a level of financial self sufficiency that will sustain the organization beyond the initial five year plan, (c) impact resident families' lives in a positive way through the delivery of individualized services, and (d) ensure client satisfaction in the form of retained management contracts from owners and surveys from owners' tenants under our control.

EHPC's model of *directly* linking housing and support services is an effective vehicle to attack poverty. This direct link, as opposed to casual, indirect referrals, enables EHPC staff to form the critical relationships with the families that foster their growth and enable problems to be dealt with in a proactive manner. As EHPC looks to the future it realizes the need to find different ways to create the nurturing and caring "EHPC Environment."

The important fiscal aspect that is critical to understand is that it costs EHPC over $200 per family per month to deliver its social services component in addition to approximately $450 per unit per month to maintain its properties. Tenant rents and Section 8 vouchers cover the physical maintenance costs. But resources to fund the social services component must be raised every year from charitable contributions and the public sector. While the annualized costs of these individualized support services approach $2,500 per family, this figure pales in comparison to the public costs for a family being forced into a homeless shelter at $1,800 per month (Kelly, 1994, p. 4), a child in the juvenile justice system at $2,000 per incidence (p. 8), or the birth of a premature child because of inadequate prenatal care at $1,000 per day of ICU care (p. 7).

The 38,000 families searching for decent housing in metropolitan St. Louis are a strong motivating force behind efforts to expand and replicate EHPC's program. True leverage must come from greater recognition of the link between decent housing and stable family environments. Governmental assistance for housing and for social services should be linked to serve holistic programs such as that offered by EHPC, rather than funding separate efforts, as has been the case in the past.

REFERENCES

Bryner, G. (1998). *The great American welfare reform debate: Politics and public morality.* New York: W.W. Norton & Company.

Center on Hunger, Poverty and Nutrition Policy. (1995). *Statement on key welfare reform issues: The empirical evidence.* Medford, MA: Author.

Children's Defense Fund. (1992, October). Child poverty hits 25-year high growing by nearly 1 million children in 1991. *CDF Reports*, pp. 1-3.

Children's Defense Fund. (1998, January). Key facts about U.S. children. *CDF Reports*, *19* (1), p. 18.

East-West Gateway Coordinating Council. (1972, July). *Recommendations for metropolitan St. Louis community development.*

East-West Gateway Coordinating Council. (1973, March). *Final draft, Regional housing plan for St. Louis metropolitan area.*

East-West Gateway Coordinating Council. (1996, July). *St. Louis Trends*, pp. 2-4.

Ecumenical Housing Production Corporation. (1981, June 5). *EHPC Update.* Unpublished report.

Ecumenical Housing Production Corporation. (1987, April 8). Report to EHPC Board on Property Management. pp. 1, 3. Unpublished report.

Gottman, K.W. (1980). *Ecumenical housing production corporation: a proposal to house low and moderate income families in St. Louis County.* p. 1. Unpublished report.

Gray, J. (1995, February 23). G.O.P. targeting social programs for budget cuts. *New York Times*, pp. A1, A10.

Harris, K.M. (1996). Life after welfare: Women, work and repeat dependency. *American Sociological Review, 61*, 407-426.

Jargowsky, P.A. & Wilson, W.J. (1997). *Poverty and place: Ghettos, barrios, and the American city.* New York: Russell Sage Foundation.

Kelly, M. (1994). *EHPC soft services: An analysis of value added.* Unpublished report.

Kenny, J. (1998, January 8). Program urges tenants to take leadership role. *St. Louis Review*, p. 9.

Koebel, C. T. (1997). Housing conditions of low-income families in the private, unassisted housing market in the United States. *Housing-Studies*, *12*, 2201-213.

Lawson, R. & Wilson, W.J. (1995). Poverty, social rights, and the quality of citizenship. In K. McFate, R. Lawson, & W.J. Wilson, *Poverty, inequality, and the future of social policy: Western states in the new world order* (pp. 693-714). New York: Russell Sage Foundation.

Liddell v. Bd. of Ed. of City of St. Louis, 491 F. Supp. 351. (E.D. Mo. 1980).

Salsich, P.W., Jr. (1997). Welfare reform: Is self sufficiency feasible without affordable housing? *Michigan Law and Policy Review*, *2*, 43-70.

Sanger, D.E. (1995, January 15). Republicans want to renew vision of Reagan (then redo his math). *New York Times*, p. 18.

Scarpetti, F. R. & Cylke, F. K., Jr. (1995). *Social problems: The search for solutions.* Los Angeles, CA: Roxbury Publishing Co.

Schmitz, C. L. (1995). Reframing the dialogue on female-headed single-parent families. *Affilia*, *10*, 426-441.

Schmitz, C. L. (1997). *Partners in Self-Sufficiency, Ecumenical Housing Production Corporation: Year five evaluation.* Unpublished report.

Schwartz, D. C., Bartlett, D. W., Ferlauto, R., & Hoffman. (1992). A new urban housing policy for the 1990s. *Journal of Urban Affairs*, *14*, 239-262.

U.S. Department of Housing and Urban Development. (1998, April). *Rental housing assistance–The crisis continues.*

Index

